QUANTUM PALEO

The Past Is Your Future. Take The Leap.

DR. DOUG WILLEN

Revised Second Edition

QUANTUM PALEO
The Past Is Your Future. Take The Leap.

DR. DOUG WILLEN
Published by Exhale Method Press
New York, NY
For more information, visit: https://exhalemethod.com

Printed Worldwide
First Printing 2012
First Edition 2012
Revised Second Printing 2026
Revised Second Edition 2026

11 10 9 8 7 6 5 4 3 2

ISBN: 978-0-9850527-0-6 (Paperback)
ISBN: 978-0-9850527-1-3 (Hardcover)
ISBN: 978-0-9850527-2-0 (Ebook)

Interior Book Design by Walt's Book Design
www.waltsbookdesign.com

Cover Design: Dr. Doug Willen

This book is for educational purposes only and is not intended as medical advice. Readers should consult a qualified healthcare professional before making changes to their health regimen.

For Lily and Max, whom I love more than life itself.

You are my inspiration and the net that appears every time I leap.

NOTE TO READER

Quantum Paleo was first written more than fifteen years ago.

At the time, my focus was simple: help patients lose weight, reduce inflammation, and regain control of their health through better food and better habits.

That mission has not changed.

Over the years my work has expanded, but the foundation still begins in the same place: the food we eat and the metabolic stress that slowly builds in the background of modern life.

Quantum Paleo was designed as a 21 day reset. A short, focused period where you step away from the foods and habits that drive inflammation and give your body a chance to recalibrate.

Many readers have used this program as a starting point. Some repeat the 21 day reset once or twice each year. Others use it as the foundation for long term lifestyle changes.

For this revised edition, I chose to keep the original spirit of the book intact. The principles still work.

A few small updates have been added to reflect what I have learned since the book was first written and to connect readers with additional resources available today.

If this is your first time reading Quantum Paleo, welcome.

If you are returning to it years later, welcome back.

Either way, the invitation is the same.

Give your body twenty one days.

Step away from the noise.

Eat simply. Move a little more.

Pay attention to how your body responds.

Sometimes the most powerful reset is simply removing what does not belong.

Let's begin.

Dr. Doug Willen

Continue Your Journey

Quantum Paleo was designed as a 21-day reset.

A chance to step away from the foods and habits that drive inflammation and allow your body to recalibrate.

Over the years my work has expanded beyond nutrition to include breathing, sleep, and metabolic health.

If you would like to continue exploring those tools, visit:

www.exhalemethod.com

Scan the QR code below to continue the journey.

www.exhalemethod.com

Inside you will find:

The Exhale Method Masterclass

The Breathing Gym

Apnea Unmasked

Additional resources for improving breathing, sleep, and metabolic health.

There is no finish line.

Only a practice.

TABLE OF CONTENTS

INTRODUCTION

What Are You Fighting For?

"Two roads diverged in a wood, and I took the one less traveled by, And that has made all the difference."

Robert Frost

Quantum Paleo is a program about transformation.

It begins with a shift in mindset. When the mind changes, the body can follow.

Many people approach health as a technical problem. They search for the right diet, the right workout, the right supplement. Those tools matter, but they rarely work by themselves.

Real change begins with a decision.

Quantum Paleo is built around short, focused cycles of change. The program starts with twenty one days. After that, you repeat additional rounds if needed until you reach your goal.

The physical changes take time.

But the moment that starts everything can happen instantly.

For me, that moment happened many years ago in India.

Death on My Hands:

The First and Last Breath

Mumbai, India, 1987

By the fourth day, I wanted to quit.

My body sagged against a tent pole in the sweltering humidity, skin sticky with sweat, mind restless and cynical. This was supposed to be a twenty one day workshop. One week of forced laughter. One week of crying. One week of silence. When I had read the description months earlier, it sounded profound. At twenty three, it felt like the key to something bigger.

By day four, I felt duped.

The instructor, a sharp eyed Israeli woman, had laid down the rules on day one.

"No speaking. No questions. No walking across the room. Crawl if you must. Sit. Laugh. Cry. Silence. That is your work."

Forty of us were sealed inside a bare, cushion lined room. No chairs. No tables. Just bodies shifting on the floor.

At first, people clustered together, forcing laughter that sounded like bad acting. I stayed on the sidelines, arms crossed, eyes narrowed. My inner critic went to work.

She's faking.

He looks ridiculous.

That one must be rich.

That one is lazy.

I invented elaborate stories about people I had never heard speak a single word.

By day four, my judgments had hardened into a fortress. I was a spectator, not a participant. Above it all. Or so I told myself.

The instructor saw right through me.

She strode over and hissed, "Quit."

I blinked. "What?"

"You already quit. So do us a favor and get the f#@k out of here."

Her words landed like a slap.

"I didn't quit," I said.

She leaned in, her voice sharp with pity and contempt.

"You're always on the sidelines, aren't you? Watching instead of living. Cynical. Self pitying. Transformation doesn't come from books or lectures. It comes from a decision. You have ten seconds. Jump in, or leave."

Then she turned her back.

I sat frozen, rage and shame boiling under my skin. My heart pounded. The air felt thick, syrupy.

I waited twelve seconds. Just to prove I could.

Then I crawled toward an older woman sitting cross legged across the room.

She wore a silk sari. Her face was carved with deep creases, her expression harder than stone. She looked, if possible, more bitter than I felt.

Perfect, I thought. At least she won't fake it.

I sat an arm's length away and locked onto her obsidian eyes. It felt like staring through prison glass.

My mind snapped back into judgment.

She's fat.

She's spoiled.

That necklace probably cost a fortune.

She's never exercised a day in her life.

Then she reached out.

Her hands were warm. Strong. Trembling. She wrapped them around mine and lifted them gently from my knees.

Silence.

My thoughts vanished, as if someone had pulled the plug from the wall.

For the first time, I truly saw her. Not the armor. Not the stories. Just her.

We locked eyes. Minutes passed.

Something in her face softened, almost imperceptibly, then cracked open into laughter.

Real laughter. Convulsive. Rolling through her body until her shoulders shook and her belly heaved.

I couldn't join her. Not at first. Her joy irritated me.

Why is she laughing?

Is she laughing at me?

Then I saw it.

A flash of myself decades later. Alone. Bitter. Poor. Clinging to regret.

A life unlived.

It hit me like a punch to the chest. And suddenly, it was funny.

My mouth twitched. A smile spread. Then the dam broke.

Laughter exploded out of me. Uncontrolled. Tears streamed. My body convulsed as something deep and long buried shook loose.

For ninety minutes, we laughed together. Waves rose and crashed, stripping us bare. Two souls exposed beneath decades of defense.

Then, stillness.

She drew in a deep breath. Held my hands tighter. Exhaled slowly.

Her head dropped forward.

At first, I thought she was resting. Then I knew she wasn't.

The instructor appeared, pressed two fingers to her neck, and shook her head once.

"She's gone," she said.

Gone.

Dead in my hands.

Her name was Niyati. Fate. Destiny.

She had come here to die. And she chose me, the angry, cynical young man, to hold her hands as she left this world.

Niyati had lived in isolation. Estranged from family. Suspicious of friends. Wealthy, but utterly alone.

She came to the ashram for one reason. To connect with one human being before she died. To laugh one last time.

And in ninety minutes, she did.

I sat trembling. Tears, mucus, breath pouring out of me. Death on my hands. Literally.

The first breath. The last breath. And between them, the rawest connection I had ever known.

The Cremation

Varanasi, India

Smoke from dozens of funeral pyres curled into the sky, blurring the line between earth and heaven. I stood off to the side, eyes burning from ash, incense, and grief woven into the air.

Niyati's body was stacked on a platform of logs at the edge of the Ganges, wrapped in linen, then covered with firewood for the cremation.

Niyati means fate. Destiny.

I did not know if I had found mine. I knew hers had led her here. To this river. And to me.

The rites unfolded.

Her body washed. Bound. White cloth, because she was a widow. Big toes tied together. A tilak pressed onto her forehead. Carried with feet facing south.

A priest stood in as lead mourner. She had no family.

He bathed. Circled the pyre. Chanted. Placed sesame seeds in her mouth. Poured ghee. Drew ash across the cloth. Yama. Kala. The dead.

An earthen pot shattered near her head.

The torch lowered.

The fire caught.

Bodies burn here every day, year after year. Smoke rising toward moksha. Liberation. No more returning. Not as a dog. Not as a grasshopper. Not at all.

I watched, transfixed.

I wondered if I should have taken the place of her son. Would they have let me?

In truth, I was the only family she had. If only for ninety minutes. She had arranged all of this herself. She knew she was coming to die.

Did she choose me? Or did I choose her?

We shared less than two hours, yet she shaped me as deeply as anyone I have ever loved.

I understood some things immediately.

Transformation can happen in an instant.

Love dissolves the rust around the soul. It softens regret. It frees what has been locked away.

For ninety minutes, she gave me her love. For ninety minutes, I gave her mine.

Life and death danced together. And I understood they are the same dance.

A boy, maybe eight years old, stepped beside me. Ribs showing. Bare feet dusted in ash. He watched the flames.

"Is she your mother?" he asked.

"Yes," I said.

Not because she gave birth to me.

But because when she held my hands, laughed with me, and exhaled her final breath, I was born.

The Lesson

Standing on the riverbank in Varanasi, watching the smoke rise into the sky, I understood something simple.

Life begins with a breath.

And it ends with one.

Everything in between is up to us.

Most people drift through those breaths without ever asking themselves a serious question about the direction of their life. They follow the most common road. The comfortable road. The road everyone else seems to be walking.

But occasionally something happens that forces you to stop.

A moment of loss.

A diagnosis.

A wake up call.

Or a stranger dying in your hands.

Those moments strip away illusion. They make you see your life clearly.

That day in India was one of those moments for me.

I realized that transformation does not begin with a diet plan or an exercise program. It begins with a decision.

A decision to step off the sidelines and participate in your own life.

A decision to stop drifting toward the same unhealthy future as everyone else.

A decision to fight for something that matters.

That realization eventually became the foundation for everything that followed.

My work with patients.

My understanding of health.

And ultimately the program you are about to begin.

Quantum Paleo is not simply a diet.

It is a framework for changing direction.

And every change begins with a single question.

What are you fighting for?

The Emperor's New Clothes

Remember the Hans Christian Andersen short tale, The Emperor's New Clothes? It reminds me of all my blind spots. It is hard to have clear vision in certain areas of life, especially regarding our own health. Coaching other people is often much easier than coaching ourselves.

Where are your blind spots?

Is it in your finances?

Your relationships?

Your health?

Or perhaps your body weight?

The significance of this allegory means different things to different people. When I reread the story recently, it provoked some self examination about my own blind spots regarding body weight, health, and longevity.

It is much more than an elementary children's story. It is a story about vanity, blind obedience, arrogance, conformity to the status quo, pretentiousness, social hypocrisy, and collective denial.

A synopsis I found captures the essence of the tale:

The Emperor's New Clothes is a short tale by Hans Christian Andersen about an emperor who cares for nothing but his wardrobe. He hires two weavers who promise him the finest suit of clothes made from a fabric invisible to anyone who is unfit for his position or hopelessly stupid.

The emperor cannot see the cloth himself, but pretends that he can for fear of appearing unfit for his position or being thought foolish. His ministers do the same.

When the swindlers report that the suit is finished, they dress him in mime and the emperor marches in procession before his subjects. A child in the crowd calls out that the emperor is wearing nothing at all and others take up the cry. The emperor cringes, suspecting the assertion is true, but holds himself up proudly and continues the procession.

You might think this is a stretch, using this story to teach a health lesson. The allegory can go in many directions. Collective denial could easily be compared to our small thinking about the food industry, our defense of refined carbohydrate diets, or the belief that low fat diets prevent heart disease.

I have read this story several times throughout my life. This time it made me think about my own health.

Believing what I wanted to believe was "the truth." Living under a veil of denial that allowed me to think my personal health plan was good enough. Erroneously believing that my exercise routine and eating habits were enough to overcome my own weak points.

The emperor was deceived because he wanted to believe the con men. He pretended the clothes were magnificent and real because he feared appearing foolish or unfit for his position. He wanted to look good on the outside, even though the inside was compromised.

Seeing Clearly

Have you ever had the feeling that you were not truly healthy even though your blood tests were considered "normal"?

Sometimes glowing test results create a false sense of security. If you still need to lose weight, improve your diet, and become more consistent with exercise, then the numbers alone do not tell the whole story.

Do you feel comforted knowing that your family tree may be riddled with heart disease, diabetes, cancer, arthritis, obesity, depression, or autoimmune disease?

It does not reassure me. It reminds me that there is work to do.

Jack Zipes, author of Hans Christian Andersen: The Misunderstood Storyteller, suggests that "seeing" in the tale is presented as the courage of one's convictions.

"Sight becomes insight, which, in turn, prompts action."

I love that line by Zipes.

Sight becomes insight, which in turn prompts action.

My Mother's Wake Up Call

Over the past twenty four months my mother experienced a major health scare involving her heart. She required two stents inserted into blocked coronary arteries. She was prescribed a cocktail of medications and underwent several medical procedures in a relatively short period of time.

Thankfully she recovered and her health stabilized. She also lost more than twenty five pounds and has kept it off. She never misses a workout.

Through diet and closely working with her healthcare team she was able to lower her score on the Hemoglobin A1C test into a normal range. The Hemoglobin A1C test reflects your average blood sugar level over the past two to three months. The test gauges how well you are managing diabetes and pre diabetes.

My mother used this turning point to gain insight.

Insight prompted action.

She needed to get her diet under control. She dropped the grains and adopted a Paleo diet. A Paleolithic diet can be extremely supportive for diabetic and pre diabetic patients.

My Own Blind Spot

In February of 2010 I was thinking about my mom's situation while lying on the couch weighing 205 pounds, with the TV remote balanced on my roll of belly fat. My body fat percentage was about 27 percent.

I was blind to my own blind spot.

I was rehearsing in my mind all the things I could tell my mom to reclaim her health. I was ready to suggest health tips and strategies to help her get back on track.

What I could not see was that I was on the same slippery slope myself.

I had solid advice for my patients, but I was in denial concerning my own health. I am not talking about the river in Egypt. Family joke. Da Nile.

Before I could "doctor" my mom, she called me and insisted that I schedule my long overdue comprehensive physical examination.

I agreed.

My doctor ordered a number of tests. I completed a heart stress test, routine blood work, and a 64 slice CT scan with a calcium score.

The results were upsetting.

The tests revealed early signs of plaque in my coronary arteries. Several markers in my lab work were outside the acceptable normal range. My blood pressure was considered high normal, which meant I was borderline hypertensive. I had occasional angina pain when I worked too many hours and did not get enough sleep.

This placed me in the ninetieth percentile of heart risk for my age. In other words, only ten percent of men in my age bracket were at greater risk than I was for having a heart incident.

If you had met me at that time you probably would have thought I looked in average shape for someone in his mid to late forties.

The test results were very upsetting.

I realized I was walking in my mother's footsteps. Actually, I was jogging in them.

I had the insight to know what needed to be done with my own health.

I needed to take action.

The Decision

I had always gone to the gym regularly. My routine back then was three days per week of ten to twelve minutes of cardio followed by twenty to thirty minutes of weight training.

This gave me the typical look of many forty to fifty year old men in my gym.

Strong.

Stocky.

With a fat gut.

It was a Thursday when I received the bad health report.

I decided I would start first thing Monday morning.

Do you ever do that?

I had my big wake up call. I decided what I was fighting for and I was determined to transform my life. I was fighting to prevent a future heart attack.

However, I needed a few more days to eat my favorite foods, polish off the ice cream in the freezer, and drink some beer in front of ESPN one more time before starting this monumental journey.

I gained two pounds that weekend while mentally preparing for my transformation.

A few things were different this time. I had said that before. But this time I was scared.

I felt it was possible that I could be facing a heart incident in the next five to ten years.

I was not ready to die.

But I also could not live with my blind spot anymore.

I hated the part of myself that made excuses and lived inauthentically.

I wrote down a list of the things I was fighting for and decided to read them every day.

I also wrote down my first goal and deadline for weight loss.

190 pounds by March 26, 2010.

My birthday.

I am fighting for:

My life.

My children Max and Lily.

My parents.

Last but not least, I wanted to look good in a bathing suit.

ROUND 1

WHAT ARE YOU FIGHTING FOR?

My birthday was nineteen days away. I decided to use my birthday as the end date for Round One.

On the morning of my birthday I was nine pounds lighter.

I was a little disappointed because I thought I might lose more weight during Round One. I decided I would repeat another round.

My birthday landed on a Friday. I needed another round to continue toward my goal weight.

I would start Round Two the following Monday morning.

I call the time between rounds

The Gap

The Gap can be challenging, so be careful.

I did not gain any weight over the Gap weekend. I worked too hard to allow myself to revert back to old habits. I read and reread my index card with my goals. This helped keep me focused.

The Gap is a time to test the concept of moderation.

The definition of moderation is the avoidance of excess or extremes, especially in one's behavior.

I want my patients to learn how to live and function with moderation, especially during times when they are not following a strict regimen.

The Quantum Paleo program is only successful if someone learns how to live and stay healthy during their normal routine.

Round One Results

I totally changed my workouts for Round One.

I began doing three forty five minute spin classes per week on Monday, Wednesday, and Friday during my lunch break, along with fifteen minutes of weight lifting.

In addition I attended a one hour boot camp training class on Tuesdays and Thursdays before work.

It was not until twelve months later that I discovered CrossFit as my preferred system of training. That story comes later in the book.

Nutritionally I incorporated the Quantum Paleo program.

My body started to visibly change. My belly was no longer protruding. My face became thinner. My entire body became stronger.

Round Two was easier than Round One. I knew my sugar cravings would disappear within forty eight to seventy two hours after quitting sugar. It takes only two to three days to get back on track.

I lost another nine pounds for a total of eighteen pounds in two rounds.

I was extremely happy with these results.

I weighed 189 pounds and held it there.

When I returned to my doctor my cholesterol dropped from 286 to 194. My triglycerides dropped from 200 to 145. My LDL came down from 130 to 98. My HDL increased from 42 to 51.

My blood pressure improved from 138 over 92 to 118 over 74.

My belly was flat and my lab work returned to the normal range.

My body fat percentage dropped to 19.5 percent.

I maintained 189 pounds easily for the entire year simply by eating Paleo.

Courage

I identify with the emperor in Andersen's story.

I see what I want to see and hear what I want to hear.

But it takes courage to see oneself authentically. It takes courage to turn sight into insight and then allow that insight to launch us into action.

The child in the story did not have the social filter that adults wear.

He simply blurted out the obvious.

"The Emperor is wearing nothing at all."

Most of what we have to do to help ourselves is obvious.

Regarding my own health I was like the emperor, believing what I wanted to believe.

In my practice I often play the role of the child, pointing out the obvious.

You need to lose weight.

You need to stop eating junk.

You should go Paleo.

You need to make the following changes and start building your health now.

If you could parade your authentic self in front of someone who had the clarity and vision of a child, what do you think they would tell you?

What feedback would you give yourself?

I am not talking about medications.

I am talking about the plan of getting back on track and producing astonishing results.

Start with this profound life changing question.

What are you fighting for?

Write it down on an index card.

Then write down the reasons that motivate you.

Fold it in half and put it in your pocket.

Read it every morning.

Read it every night.

Do not wait.

Do it now.

ROUND 2

WHAT IS PALEO?

The word "Paleo" refers to the term "Paleolithic," which was coined by the archaeologist John Lubbock in 1865. The word derives from the Greek terms palaios, meaning old, and lithos, meaning stone. It literally translates to "old stone age."

Today the word Paleo is commonly used to describe a grain free style of eating.

The Stone Age, or Paleolithic era, occurred from roughly 2.5 million years ago until about 10,000 years ago. During that time our ancestors survived by hunting and gathering food from their environment.

Agriculture did not exist yet. Farming did not exist yet. Processed food certainly did not exist yet.

Our ancestors ate what they could hunt, catch, or gather.

Modern agriculture, by contrast, has only existed for approximately the last 10,000 years. That may sound like a long time. In evolutionary terms, it is only a brief moment.

More than 99 percent of your genetic blueprint was formed long before agriculture appeared. In other words, your genetic makeup is virtually identical to that of your Paleolithic ancestors.

Your genetic code was shaped over millions of years. That means certain foods and nutrients, the same ones your ancient biological ancestors consumed, are literally part of your biology today.

Good health can be expected when you feed your body the foods to which it has genetically adapted. Conversely, when we feed our bodies foods that we have not adapted to, dyspepsia, degeneration, and disease will follow.

In 1985 Dr. Boyd Eaton of Emory University in Atlanta wrote a landmark paper titled Paleolithic Nutrition, which was published in the prestigious New England Journal of Medicine. The basic premise of that report was simple.

Our genes determine our nutritional needs.

For millions of years humans ate what they could hunt and gather. Today many people eat what looks good, tastes good, or what is sold to them through multi million dollar advertising campaigns.

The average American now consumes roughly 150 pounds of sugar and sweeteners every year, along with hundreds of pounds of grain based foods.

That dramatic shift away from our evolutionary diet has consequences.

Medical doctor James Braly and researcher Ron Hoggan wrote a book titled Dangerous Grains. Their research documents how grain consumption is linked to more than two hundred chronic illnesses and conditions.

These include Type 2 diabetes, cancer, heart disease, arthritis, autoimmune diseases, brain disorders, intestinal diseases, chronic pain, infertility, and problematic pregnancies, to name only a few.

Our hunter gatherer ancestors, by contrast, were typically lean, strong, and physically capable. They survived on animal proteins such as meat, fish, and fowl along with fruits, vegetables, nuts, seeds, and healthy natural fats.

Dairy and starches were only available intermittently. Livestock had not yet been domesticated, so regular access to milk producing animals did not exist.

Root vegetables and naturally occurring starches were gathered rather than planted and farmed in large quantities.

Items that needed to be hunted or gathered were not always available on a consistent basis. Availability depended on geography, season, and the success of the hunt.

Grains and refined sugar were not available during the Paleolithic era. People living during that time did not have access to bread, pasta, and the many grain based foods that dominate the modern diet.

Interestingly, the degenerative diseases that plague modern society were also largely absent.

The Paleo way of eating attempts to match modern nutrition with the foods that human beings are genetically designed to eat. When people follow this approach, they often experience dramatic improvements in their health, energy, and body composition.

In my own practice I have seen patients successfully turn back the clock to a time in their lives when they were not constantly tired or struggling with their weight.

It is exciting to watch people reclaim their health and return to a natural body weight.

What Are the Benefits of Going Paleo?

There are numerous benefits that people can experience by switching to a Paleo style of eating.

In my practice I repeatedly see several common improvements.

Weight Loss

Many people lose between 6 and 18 pounds during the first 21 days of the program.

I once conducted a corporate team building event based on the Quantum Paleo program. Two teams of twenty employees competed in a 21 day challenge.

The results were remarkable.

One participant, Bryan, lost 26 pounds.

Another participant, Larry, lost 22 pounds.

Dave lost 18 pounds.

Six others lost between 13 and 16 pounds.

Our top female competitor lost 15 pounds in just three weeks.

Three additional women lost between 9 and 12 pounds.

These results were achieved in only 21 days.

Health Improvements

The list of possible health improvements is extensive.

Most people report increased energy and lower stress levels within the first few days.

Improvements often occur in multiple systems of the body including immune function, digestion, and musculoskeletal health.

Each person's experience is different, but the pattern is consistent. When people remove problematic foods and begin eating real food again, the body often responds quickly.

Better Sleep

Removing refined carbohydrates, sugars, trans fats, junk food, and chemical additives from the diet often results in improved sleep.

Improved Sex Drive

When people lose weight and begin to feel better about their bodies, libido often improves as well. Partners frequently notice the difference.

Longevity

Eating foods that match our biological design supports long term health and vitality.

Strength and Fitness

Many high performing athletes now follow nutrition programs that closely resemble Paleo style eating.

Grains: The Good, The Bad, and The Ugly

Many common grains such as wheat, rye, and barley contain compounds that can irritate the digestive tract and trigger immune reactions.

Three key terms that frequently appear in discussions about grains are gluten, lectins, and phytates.

Gluten

Gluten is the protein found in wheat and several other grains. It gives dough its elastic structure.

Gluten is made up of two primary proteins called gliadin and glutenin.

Research suggests that the human ability to digest gluten may be decreasing. Some researchers, including those at the Mayo Clinic, report that gluten related sensitivities appear to be becoming more common.

Celiac Disease

Celiac disease is an autoimmune disorder affecting the small intestine.

Approximately 1 percent of the population has celiac disease.

Symptoms may include chronic diarrhea, fatigue, poor growth in children, and nutrient deficiencies.

When individuals with celiac disease consume gluten, their immune system attacks the lining of the small intestine. This damages the intestinal villi, the structures responsible for absorbing nutrients.

When the villi are damaged, nutrient absorption becomes impaired, which can lead to malnutrition and other health complications.

Celiac disease is frequently underdiagnosed. Some estimates suggest that for every diagnosed patient, many more remain undiagnosed.

In addition, millions of people may experience non celiac gluten sensitivity, meaning they react poorly to gluten without having full celiac disease.

Lectins and Phytates

Plants have a built in self defense mechanism that they rely on for survival. For a plant to reproduce, it must rely on outside sources to spread its seeds. Sometimes it is the wind. Sometimes birds and insects help spread the seeds.

The plant cannot generate movement in order to spread its own seed to ensure its survival. Therefore, it has several methods to help the seed survive long enough for it to implant in soil at a distance from the original plant.

Grains produce compounds such as lectins and phytates. These are toxic substances that act as anti nutrients. An anti nutrient literally prevents the body from absorbing certain vitamins and minerals by disrupting absorption.

These compounds are poisonous to insects, birds, and even humans, and make it very difficult for them to digest the entire seed or nut. The seed or nut will often be safely passed or defecated back into the earth.

Fruits are an exception because they are not anti nutrients and do not pose the same danger as grains. When an animal eats fruit, the seeds pass through and exit the body. This is a perfect design in nature. The seed survives because the seed is indigestible.

Some animals have clearly adapted to grain consumption. Birds, rodents, and some insects can deal with the anti nutrients. Humans, however, cannot.

Three Whites for 90 Days

There is a quote from Nancy Appleton's book Lick the Sugar Habit that I both love and hate.

"80 percent of sick people would get well if they eliminated dairy, wheat, and sugar."

I love that quote because it is probably true.

I hate that quote because it is probably true.

For years I have told my patients to eliminate what I call the three whites.

Sugar.

Flour.

Dairy.

I do not enjoy telling people to eliminate these foods.

But I have seen the results too many times to ignore.

When people remove these foods, sick people often get better.

Chronically overweight people who struggled for years often begin losing weight.

I once treated a patient named Stan who worked as a restaurant chef.

His hands were his livelihood.

At age forty four he could no longer close his hands around a chef's knife.

His fingers were swollen and painful. His joints were inflamed. His knees, ankles, elbows, and shoulders hurt constantly.

His muscles ached throughout his back, neck, hips, chest, and legs.

His physician diagnosed him with arthritis and fibromyalgia.

We ran a series of tests including an IgG food sensitivity test and blood work.

IgG food sensitivity test

The results showed that he reacted strongly to grains, sugar, and dairy. He also showed signs of gluten sensitivity.

I told him to eliminate the three whites for ninety days.

That meant removing grains, dairy, and sugar completely.

He committed to the Quantum Paleo program.

Six weeks later he returned to my office pain free.

The swelling and redness in his hands had disappeared. His fibromyalgia symptoms were gone.

At the end of the ninety days Stan had lost thirty six pounds.

He tried reintroducing bread and pasta into his diet.

Within hours the pain and swelling returned.

That was enough to convince him.

He stayed with the diet long term.

Whenever I am unsure how to help someone struggling with chronic illness, I start by cleaning up the diet.

Remove the grains.

Remove the sugar.

Remove the dairy.

Start with the gut

A professor of mine used to say, "Start with the gut and you can never go wrong."

If you have a chronic condition, especially one involving inflammation, consider the possibility that food is a critical piece of the puzzle.

Try eliminating the three whites and see what happens.

The Paleo diet was a new term for me when I first encountered it.

But the idea was not new.

For more than a decade I had been recommending essentially the same approach to my patients.

Back then I simply called it the hunter gatherer diet.

Or even simpler.

Eliminate the three whites

For ninety days.

That simple approach built my entire practice.

Today people call it Paleo.

Some call it Primal.

Others call it the Caveman diet.

The name does not matter.

As Shakespeare wrote,

"A rose by any other name would smell as sweet."

ROUND 3

QUANTUM PALEO

What is *Quantum Paleo*? What does it mean? How is it different than what others are teaching, writing, and blogging about concerning this subject?

That was a question I was asked when I started writing this book.

My point of view is what makes this program unique. This book is different because I come from a clinical background. I am not a biochemist, anthropologist, or an elite athlete who has adopted this way of life.

I have put thousands of people on grain free diets in the past fourteen years. I have always used a grain free program. Not because it closely resembles the diet of our Paleolithic ancestors. Fourteen years ago I had never even heard the term Paleo. I put people on grain free diets because it got sick people well. Period. I also took people off sugar and dairy. It helped people reclaim their lost health.

Quantum Paleo is a book that includes the mindset needed to succeed. In my clinical experience I have worked with many people who need support not only with the "how to," but also the "why." Quantum Paleo drills down to the soul and gut level, enabling people to make lasting changes.

I am excited to read the informative blogs and books on this subject. There is a whole world of Paleo people in the online community today. I am even more excited to understand the reason that sick people get well on a grain free diet. The Paleo way of eating is the only diet that closely matches what we can eat according to our genetic makeup and evolutionary development.

Great. We have an extraordinary diet. We even have historical, anthropological, and evolutionary reasons to dial into this life changing information. However, in the past fourteen years I have often run into a stonewall with patients when trying to get them to stick with the program long enough to see results. If people do not have a crystal clear goal of what they are fighting for, they may not succeed.

I eventually challenged my patients to incorporate the "why" into their goal setting. I found that when patients wrote down their goals and answered the question of what they were fighting for, their results with chronic health conditions improved dramatically. Their resolve strengthened. Patients who did this basic exercise tended to stick with the regimen long enough to see results.

Most of us do not choose to eat foods for the same reasons our Paleolithic ancestors did. Our Paleolithic great aunts and uncles did not have the temptation of a breadbasket being placed on the table every time they went to a restaurant. They did not have to stare down a pizza or birthday cake and resist the urge to take a bite.

I would be willing to bet that if you offered a caveman a seat on your couch, an overstuffed sandwich, and a beer while watching a Sunday afternoon football game, he probably would not turn you down.

We live in a time where many of us eat primarily for pleasure. We emotionally select our foods without thinking about survival. Paleolithic people probably experienced tremendous joy when eating their favorite foods as well. The crucial difference was that their primary concern was survival.

How does a person living today avoid all of the tempting, delicious foods and choose correctly? Are we supposed to avoid pizza for the rest of our lives?

These are relevant and appropriate questions. My approach is to commit to a short period of time and get healthy as fast as possible. To do this you must follow the program with focus and intensity. Learn your body's nutritional needs so it can function and express health at its highest potential. Then make wise choices to maintain lasting health.

I have shown patients their blood work and supporting research that clearly proves they must change their diet. Yet some still struggle to comply and stay the course even when facing serious symptoms, conditions, or disease.

Have you ever seen someone who had throat cancer surgery, where the surgeon leaves a small hole in their windpipe to breathe and talk? I have seen throat cancer survivors remove their scarf and take a drag off a cigarette through the hole in their neck. They know they must quit. Yet they still smoke through the hole in their windpipe.

That person never had the mental shift needed to transform their life.

I feel their healthcare is incomplete. They may have had a successful surgery, but no one addressed the mindset. The person never experienced the breakthrough at the soul level.

I have been face to face with people who need to change and want to change, but still do not.

My approach is what I call Quantum Paleo. This program not only addresses diet, exercise, and lifestyle, but it also helps uncover the beliefs and hang ups that hold people back.

I also realize there may be people reading this book who do not need motivation or guidance. They start a new program and immediately gain momentum as the weeks go by. They are strong, athletic, and have the willpower to make dramatic changes with very little guidance. If you are one of those people, then use this book as a quick guide.

Most of my patients over the years need more than motivation, inspirational quotes, diet menus, and weigh ins to achieve success. I push my patients to dig down and find the limiting factor that is holding them back. They need to tap into something worth fighting for. It can only be found at a core level.

When a patient finds the core reason to change, it is extremely emotional. I have seen patients break out in tears. It must be something truly personal. It must touch their soul.

Next I pull on that thread and slowly unravel the fear, insecurity, and regret that often accompany someone who has struggled with their health and body for years.

It takes a personal leap away from the current traditional American way of eating to arrive at a new place of health and longevity.

Quantum Paleo is the program that can take you there.

Religiousness

The more I read about how Paleolithic eating is interpreted, the more confused I get. Some people write that to be Paleo you can never eat this or that. Others loosely define the parameters of what constitutes a Paleo program, while some are downright zealots.

The real extremists are almost ready to trade their jeans, T shirt, and credit cards for a loincloth and a spear. I call them Paleo Evangelists.

I am not ready to give up a cup of ice cream every once in a while. I also want to try my share of local and foreign beers throughout my life.

Beer, by the way, is not Paleo.

What a conundrum.

I also like chocolate. How about you?

I started with all this Paleo work in my practice fourteen years ago trying to help sick people get well. The people calling for appointments were not healthy athletes or CrossFit enthusiasts. They were not even healthy. They were chronically ill people, and the word Paleo was not even on my radar at the time.

I was taught by my nutrition professor to take patients off the three whites, dairy, sugar, and grains, and eighty percent of them would get well.

At first I did not believe that changing the way people eat could turn around their health. I was impressed by the results I witnessed after doing the rounds with him in his clinic and talking directly with patients about their cases. I interviewed patients with serious health issues and heard dozens of stories of how removing grains improved their health. The most impressive part was seeing their blood tests support what they were feeling in their bodies.

What is the reason we should even care about a Paleo type of diet? Is it because we secretly wish to live the simple, rustic lives of hunters and gatherers? Some people do.

As a healthcare provider I believe the mass appeal comes from the remarkable health benefits that many people experience. The ability to maintain a lean, fit body after years of failing miserably on other diets is extremely appealing.

A few years ago I heard the word Paleo for the first time. The three white elimination diet that I was using with patients was essentially the same as what is now called Paleo. Whatever you call it, it works.

If this is true, certain questions will inevitably arise.

"How strict do I have to be to get results?"

"Can I ever have a beer?"

"How about wine or a shot of tequila?"

"Pizza? Baguette? Tortilla? Crepe? Or Grandma's famous chocolate ice box ladyfinger cake passed down through generations?"

This is the point where I am sure I will get some negative comments. I am not the 100 percent guy you may be looking for. My point of view comes primarily from my role as a healthcare provider.

When I sit with a patient and evaluate the severity of their symptoms and conditions, I recommend how strictly they should follow the diet. If their health is seriously compromised, I recommend they follow the program at 100 percent for at least ninety days.

No cheating. Full commitment.

Then we reevaluate how they are feeling at that point. Throughout this process I help them move toward a lifelong transition to the Paleo mindset.

In my practice I also use a blood test called the IgG Food Sensitivity Test. I have used this test for almost fifteen years. It helps identify how reactive dairy, grains, sugar, and many other foods are for a patient.

IgG Food Sensitivity Test

If the patient completes the ninety days and their test results show improvement, I allow them to experiment cautiously with occasional foods such as ice cream or a beer.

Whether they can maintain results while occasionally enjoying these foods depends on their ability to maintain balance in the body. That is my perspective.

I am strict in the beginning.

Later we experiment carefully with occasional treats.

The definition of the word food is any nutritious substance that people or animals eat or drink in order to maintain life and growth.

The definition of the word treat is something out of the ordinary that gives pleasure.

According to that definition, ice cream is not food.

Ice cream is a treat.

We do not need treats every day. They are the exception, not the routine. This is crucially important.

Ice cream, beer, and bread are treats and should not be consumed every day. If your body can tolerate them occasionally, then enjoy them as treats.

These days I work with many healthy people who are excited to adopt a new way of living. Many are young, athletic, and symptom free individuals who already understand the Paleo mindset. With these people we talk about balance.

To maintain an elite level of vitality and health, your diet must be on target.

Can you have an occasional beer night?

I want you to.

We are not living in the Paleolithic era. There are many enjoyable foods and drinks available. Staying in balance is the challenge.

Greg Glassman, founder of CrossFit, once said that many people approach Paleo eating the same way they approach religious rules.

He explained that some people become almost fanatical about every ingredient they consume, worrying whether something is Paleo or not.

The point is that any diet, Paleo, Zone, or otherwise, should ultimately support human health and performance.

Your focus should be on improving your health and performance, not on winning a contest about who eats the most perfect diet.

One way to take Paleo up a notch is by controlling calorie intake and portion sizes. I often combine a Paleo style diet with an initial period of calorie restriction.

The real question is why you are doing a Paleo diet in the first place.

Are you trying to get healthy?

Are you trying to look good naked?

Are you trying to improve athletic performance?

All of these are valid reasons.

Some people attempt to recreate the exact diet of a caveman. That is not what I teach.

My goal is simple. I want results for my patients.

The Paleo way of eating is superior to many other approaches.

We start with an initial stage of eliminating grains, sugar, and dairy completely.

After that we learn what the body can tolerate.

Some people may tolerate small amounts occasionally.

Others may learn they can never eat grains and remain healthy.

That is the reality.

I encourage patients to follow the program strictly for at least twenty one days so they can experience its full potential.

Then they can decide what works best for their own body.

Is Paleo Unhealthy?

Are Paleo diets unhealthy?

No.

I have been teaching and implementing a Paleo style diet in my practice for more than fourteen years.

Tuesday night group workshop in NYC reference

Whenever I introduced this program I heard the same questions.

"Is it unhealthy to eliminate grains?"

"What will I have left to eat?"

"If I eat protein, vegetables, healthy fats, some fruit, seeds, nuts, and water, will that hurt me?"

Some people even told me they needed to check with their regular doctor before trying such a radical diet.

I have had people demand refunds from my classes after asking their doctor whether this diet was healthy. Their doctor told them that grain free diets were unhealthy, foolish, and unscientific.

My response at the time was simple.

"What a load of woolly mammoth crap."

Let this sink in. The Paleo way of eating closely matches the foods our genetics evolved to process.

Our genetic code determines our nutritional needs.

The following is a short list of conditions that have improved or resolved in my practice over the past fourteen years:

- Malabsorption
- Gastritis

- Colitis
- Chronic Diarrhea
- Flatulence
- Delayed Menarche
- Liver Disease
- Leaky Gut Syndrome
- Impotence
- Low Libido
- Iron Deficiency Anemia
- IBS
- Kidney Disease
- Heart Disease
- Type 2 Diabetes
- Grave's Disease
- Alopecia
- Nausea
- Vomiting
- Bloating
- Ulcerative Colitis
- Chronic Fatigue
- Eczema
- Edema
- ADD/ADHD
- Autism
- Schizophrenia
- Anxiety
- Epilepsy
- Failure to Thrive
- Gastrointestinal Bleeding

- Cerebral Atrophy
- Celiac Disease
- Chest Pain
- Cancer
- Bladder Cancer
- Brain Cancer
- Prostate Cancer
- Osteoporosis
- Autoimmune Diseases
- Lupus
- Ataxia
- Hyperthyroidism
- Miscarriages
- Amenorrhea
- Arthritis
- Fibromyalgia
- Oral Cancers
- Multiple Sclerosis
- Trigeminal Neuritis
- Myasthenia Gravis
- Infertility
- Still Births
- Otitis Media
- Pancreatitis
- Depression
- Osteomalacia
- Rheumatoid Arthritis
- Delayed Puberty
- Eczema

- Hives
- Weight Loss
- PMS
- Improved Hemoglobin A1C Scores
- Psoriasis
- Hypothyroidism
- Vitiligo

This is not simply a list of conditions I have read about in books. These are results from cases I personally monitored in patients who adopted a Paleo way of eating.

Expect it may take three to twelve months to transform your health and body. Some people will be satisfied to see their symptoms improve. Others will experience life changing results.

What is possible?

The Quantum Paleo program can take you back to reclaiming your body.

Do not make it complicated. This book is about gaining the vision to make a change. The most important step is simply getting started. Keep it simple.

"Whatever the mind can conceive and believe, the mind can achieve."

Dr. Napoleon Hill.

ROUND 4

THE CHALLENGE

I call this the Challenge Section because it will challenge you to think, plan, feel, and take action. This is the section that separates my book from other Paleo books. I have worked with thousands of patients over the last 14 years. I have seen many people frustrated with their inability to lose weight and reclaim their health. Over time, I created a program to help people take a quantum leap toward attaining the success that has eluded them in the past. I will share with you the tools I extracted from years in the trenches helping the most stubborn cases succeed.

Health: Is It Definable?

Many people define "health" as the state of "not being sick." I think "not being sick" is a lousy definition of health.

Dorland's Medical Dictionary defines health as:

"a state of optimal physical, mental and social wellbeing, and not merely the absence of disease and infirmity."

I like Dorland's definition. It works for me.

Health is a work in progress. Defining health is as challenging and elusive as trying to define a river. I picture the concept of health as having the shape, body, and characteristics of a river. A river is ever changing. It is never the same from moment to moment. Our bodies have many variables that affect our physical, mental, and social well-being. For example: age, stress, personal finances, physical conditioning, disease, infection, prescription medication, work responsibilities, diet, levels of macro and micronutrients, work conditions, quality of sleep, and hydration. The list could be extensive.

I think the key insight is that all the categories are essential: physical, mental, and social well-being.

I have worked with many elite level athletes over the years. Most elite athletes enjoy superior health. I can recall a few elite athletes who were not truly healthy in all areas. Gerry, 27 years old, was one patient who fit this profile. On one hand, she could claim she was never sick a day in her life. At the same time, she was in an abusive marriage filled with anger, hate, resentment, humiliation, and shame. She clearly did not fit Dorland's Medical Dictionary definition of health. She booked an exam and consultation to determine if changing her diet would add to her health.

I performed a complete history and exam. I also checked her with my Nutritional Kinesiology technique, along with another kinesiology approach that works on the emotional connection to illness.

Bingo. Her emotional points were particularly active, especially the grief and anger points. I shared my findings, which must have struck a deep chord because she burst into tears. She could not stop sobbing. Now the whole story came out. She told me she was trapped in a horrible marriage. Her husband was abusive both physically and verbally. The verbal and mental abuse was happening daily.

She only came in for about half a dozen sessions.

I gave her a few chiropractic adjustments and tweaked her diet slightly. She was already following a Paleo diet. Over those few sessions she told me her story one piece at a time.

I encouraged her to get support to help address her marriage and relationship issues. I saw her again about a year later, and she told me the marriage had ended in divorce. At that point I felt she was truly healthy.

Now she had the mental and social well-being components in place that are critical to overall health.

If your goal for health is bragging about all the days you are not sick, you are limiting yourself. We all need to raise the bar. Aim for a higher goal. Striving for optimal physical, mental, and social well-being is a worthy goal.

You cannot buy health or own it. We only rent it. Hopefully it is a long-term lease. It requires regular payments and upkeep. If you neglect your health, it may rapidly erode. It comes down to seeing the big picture. Decide what is important to you, then fight for it.

What Did You Feed the Dog?

How to feel good from the inside out

So much of how we feel and heal is determined by what we put into our bodies. The foods we eat can lead to health and vitality. Conversely, they can lead to chronic illness, allergies, asthma, skin problems, insomnia, low libido, digestive issues, headaches, hormonal imbalance, exacerbation of autoimmune conditions, and even pain and inflammation in our joints.

It amazes me how often people disconnect the foods they eat from how their bodies function. My patients come in and report multiple symptoms that are preventing them from fully enjoying their lives.

When I suggest they need to get their diet right, I often hear questions such as, "Do you think food could be playing a role?" or "My doctor said the foods I eat have nothing to do with the fact that I have diarrhea 11 times per day."

When our family dog has terrible skin, poops on the floor, has diarrhea, retreats to her bed, and stays curled up in a ball all day, we automatically ask each other one question. What did you feed the dog?

Or we ask, "Did the dog get into the garbage again?"

Why?

Because what goes into the dog's mouth has a lot to do with what comes out the other end.

What goes into the dog has a lot to do with the health of the dog.

Why would that logic not apply to us as well?

We have perfect clarity when it comes to babies. Most people would never put cola or root beer in a baby's bottle. Of course not. How about a shot of whiskey in the baby bottle, or some chewing tobacco between the cheek and gum? How about artificial flavorings, preservatives, food dyes, and colors, topped off with a few teaspoons of sugar or salt?

If you saw someone feeding a baby this way, would you say something? Maybe that would feel too confrontational. But we could all agree it would be shocking to witness.

Would you expect such behavior to cause health problems?

It might cause swelling, bloating, diarrhea, poor sleep, digestive issues, failure to thrive, rapid heartbeat, mood swings, attention problems, depression, lethargy, or hyperactivity. In other words, a chronically sick baby.

This is where we see the big blind spot.

We see it clearly with the dog.

We see it clearly with the baby.

Why can't we see it in ourselves?

Every day in my office I hear people say, "I can't believe the foods I choose could have that much to do with my health and emotional state."

How old does the baby need to be before we feel it is acceptable to feed that same human being junk food? At some point it becomes socially acceptable to feed the human body this way.

Before six months, one year, or even two years old, it might be considered abuse. At what age does it suddenly become normal, socially acceptable, and even healthy?

Are you chronically tired and getting sick too often? Are your hormones out of balance? Are you feeling down, and is your libido lower than whale turd on the bottom of the ocean? Then it may be time to clean up your act.

Quantum Paleo is effective because as you lose weight you also clean up the small health problems that accumulate with age. Aging is real. To a greater extent than most people realize, we choose how we age.

If you stick with Quantum Paleo for 21 days, you will begin to lose weight and feel fantastic. Your emotional state will begin to balance.

The best test is to commit to a 21 day trial.

What if you were the success story at the back of the book?

How would that change your life?

Challenge #1

Here is your first challenge. Take out your journal or notebook and write down your success story before you start the Quantum Paleo program. I am serious. Make it up. Invent it.

Crazy idea? Not really.

What if you wrote down everything you want to change as if it already happened?

Here is an example of what that might look like. This is an actual journal entry from a patient who tried this exercise before starting the Quantum Paleo program. Everything in this prediction came true except that she lost 13.2 pounds in 21 days rather than the 11.5 pounds she predicted.

Here is the journal entry.

"Dear Dr. Doug,

Not only did I lose 11.5 pounds in 21 days, but my body has never felt better. I am pooping every day like clockwork. I feel recharged in the mornings after a good night's sleep. I am exercising with purpose. My cholesterol and triglycerides are now in the normal range. My Hemoglobin A1c is normal too. Did I mention my sex life? Oh boy has that changed. My libido is better than it has been in 15 years.

In the last few days I started dreaming and planning my future. I want to go back to school and finish my certification so I can earn more money. I am playing the guitar again. I have so many plans and goals swimming in my head.

People at work are noticing too. They want to know my secret.

One of the biggest shifts was patching things up with my dad. I was certain he would shoot me down when I approached him. It was nothing like I expected. To make a long story short, we are reconnecting.

The funny thing is I find myself with better willpower when I am not at war with people in my life. Is that possible?

I am going to take two days off and then start another round. Next goal: looking great in a bathing suit for the summer.

Thanks Dr. D!"

Write down your results before they happen. Write exactly how you want your future to unfold. It takes imagination. It may feel ridiculous. Try it. Have the courage. What do you have to lose?

Challenge #2

Okay. That's the body. What about the mind?

I want you to bring back an old hobby that you have not done in years. It might be knitting, horseback riding, singing in the shower, or playing that old guitar you have not touched in years. Maybe photography, watercolor painting, or even finger painting. Maybe something outdoors like hiking, frisbee, or tennis.

Start doing something creative or enjoyable again. It sends a message to yourself that you are worth it.

Before I created the Quantum Paleo program, I used to supervise a 21 day cleanse or detox diet with my patients either in person or over the phone. I have been doing it for more than 14 years. This eventually became the workshop and support group I taught every Tuesday night in New York City for three years.

It was first called the *Eliminate the 3 Whites Diet*, then it changed to the *Purification Diet*, and eventually I called it *The Big Sweep*.

I always worked in rounds of 21 days. The main difference between the Purification Diet and the Quantum Paleo program was that I gave my patients herbal supplements designed to help cleanse and detoxify their bodies. It became a very popular workshop. I eventually stopped teaching it so I could spend more time at home with my kids.

Everyone lost weight, symptoms improved, and people watched their health improve dramatically. My guidelines were simple: follow the diet and try something creative or fun that would bring you joy.

My favorite part of the evening was when participants shared the hobbies and creative pursuits they had brought back into their lives.

One woman in the cleanse group, Clarice, was caring for her terminally ill husband. They were retired and could not afford a home nurse. She cared for him 24 hours per day for almost a year. She was completely consumed with taking care of him and never made time to do anything enjoyable for herself.

She followed the diet program diligently, but she insisted she had no time to experiment with my suggestion of incorporating a hobby or creative outlet. She could not remember the last time she even smiled.

One night she shared with the group that years earlier she had enjoyed memorizing poems and occasionally reciting them to friends. This used to make her happy.

We all encouraged her to bring a poem into class the following week. She agreed to memorize one and recite it to us.

The next class she recited a poem by Robert Frost.

Stopping by Woods on a Snowy Evening

by Robert Frost

Whose woods these are I think I know.

His house is in the village, though;

He will not see me stopping here

To watch his woods fill up with snow.

My little horse must think it queer

To stop without a farmhouse near

Between the woods and frozen lake

The darkest evening of the year.

He gives his harness bells a shake

To ask if there is some mistake.

The only other sounds the sweep

Of easy wind and downy flake.

The woods are lovely, dark, and deep,

But I have promises to keep,

And miles to go before I sleep,

And miles to go before I sleep.

She spoke with such passion, totally transported. I felt goosebumps immediately and was transfixed by her eyes as they began to tear up halfway through the passage.

Thirty-two of us were all sniffling and teary. Not so much from the poem itself, but from the miracle of transformation we were witnessing. When she finished, the room was absolutely quiet for about thirty seconds. Then we all jumped up to give her hugs and share our reactions.

It was amazing that she chose that poem. For me, the last stanza is about responsibility. I love this poem. Of course, you may see it differently than I do. The poem has always made me aware of the juxtaposition between pausing in life to appreciate something simple and beautiful, and the constant pull to return to our work and carry through with our obligations.

Her hard, wooden, emotionless face softened that night. We saw her transform right in front of our eyes. In a way, we transformed with her.

Remember, health is not merely the absence of disease. It is a balance of physical, mental, and social well-being.

To feel good, you need to look on the inside. You will only scratch the surface if your goal is simply to start and finish the 21-day Quantum Paleo program.

Branch out and look for ways to bring some fun back into your life. Restart a hobby or begin a project that will bring you joy.

If you made it this far in the book, then you probably had a thought or an idea pop into your head when I mentioned a creative pursuit or hobby. This may be something sitting quietly in a forgotten corner of your past.

Here is your chance to dust it off and bring it back into your life. Go to my website and share with me in the Success Stories section what activity you are bringing back into your life. Sharing can inspire and act as a catalyst of transformation for someone else. Do not be stingy. Passively reading this book is not nearly as powerful as actively participating.

The Man in the Arena

Excerpt from the speech *Citizenship In A Republic*, delivered by Theodore Roosevelt at the Sorbonne in Paris, France, on April 23, 1910.

"It is not the critic who counts; not the man who points out how the strong man stumbles, or where the doer of deeds could have done them better. The credit belongs to the man who is actually in the arena, whose face is marred by dust and sweat and blood; who strives valiantly; who errs, who comes short again and again, because there is no effort without error and shortcoming; but who does actually strive to do the deeds; who knows great enthusiasms, the great devotions; who spends himself in a worthy cause; who at the best knows in the end the triumph of high achievement, and who at the worst, if he fails, at least fails while daring greatly, so that his place shall never be with those cold and timid souls who neither know victory nor defeat."

This may be my all-time favorite quote. The credit belongs to the person who participates, who takes on the challenge, and fights for something worth fighting for. You must try and try again regardless of the outcome. Either way, you will never be among those cold and timid souls who know neither victory nor defeat.

My personal challenge is to stay in the arena. I have failed at many things. I have struggled with managing my finances, my career, my health, and my body weight. That is what the Quantum Paleo program is about. The program is a way of life. I could have called it the *Fight For The Life You Want Diet*, but that did not sound nearly as catchy.

Notice that Theodore Roosevelt did not say, "The credit belongs to the person who does it perfectly," or "The credit belongs to the person with a perfect track record." He said we need to be in the arena.

Here is how to do the diet. You jump in the arena and start. Follow the plan. Be forewarned that there is always an opponent. The opponent is your temptations, your fears, your self-doubt, and your critics. This opponent wants to hold you down and make you submit and quit.

There comes a time to fight. There is a part of you that will want to quit when things get tough. You may not lose as much weight as you want the first week, or even the second week. You may find yourself constipated or gassy. Just do the 21-day program anyway.

Do not wait for perfection, because it is not coming. Do not wait for the perfect moment on the calendar to start. Do not worry if everything is not perfect.

Get in the arena and do your best.

That is all I am asking.

It will work if you do.

Live Out Loud

"I came to live out loud!"

Emile Zola

One of the reasons diets fail is that people create an escape plan before they even begin. When someone keeps their goals a secret, it becomes easy to abort the mission and return to base. They buy a round-trip ticket before the journey even begins.

They secretly plan to return to their comfortable rut as soon as they step outside of it.

Tell other people about your plans to transform your health and lose weight. This is what I call living out loud. It becomes a one-way ticket. You are essentially saying, "Once I cross that bridge, I am not coming back."

This is very different from how most people approach dieting. Most people secretly skim a diet book in a bookstore without even buying it. Then they binge over the weekend and begin the diet Monday morning. By Wednesday they have already quit.

It was so secretive and sneaky that not even their spouse knew they were attempting a diet. They might say something vague like,

"No bread today. I feel too stuffed from the weekend."

Vague, isn't it? We are not even sure if they started anything. Worst of all, they are not sure either.

This is someone dabbling with the diet. They will most likely quit within a few days. The voyage is doomed before it even leaves the harbor.

Imagine going into battle with this person.

"I got your back for a few seconds. When things get tough, I'm out of here."

Challenge #3

Decide to live out loud.

Declare that you are doing the Quantum Paleo program. Tell at least five people other than your significant other. Share your goals with people who are important in your life.

Congratulations. You just increased your chances of success by 95 percent.

The Gateway to Success

To enter the Kingdom of Success, you must first pass through a gateway. Blocking your path is the biggest opponent of all. The opponent you must face is yourself.

This next challenge is critical. It is the step most people skip. Think of it as a ritual or ceremony.

You are about to enter the Quantum Paleo arena and climb into the octagon. It is time to fight for your life and reclaim your health and body.

You are cloaked with a cape of failure as you approach the fighting cage. The cape needs to be dropped. The cape represents your fears, regrets, self-hate, and past failures.

Yes, you can skip ahead and approach this diet mechanically. But let me ask you something. Why are you not at your ideal weight right now? Why did you buy this diet book?

If you had already mastered your weight and health, you would not be reading this book.

Are you like me, riding the roller coaster of gaining and losing weight throughout your adult life? Have you been heavy for as long as you can remember? Have you tried other programs before, only to return to the same place or worse?

I am going to show you how to save time. If you complete this challenge, it will become easier to reach and maintain your ideal body weight.

The diet itself is explained in Round 7. It is not rocket science.

It is four to five meals per day, with an optional snack if needed. The diet consists of protein, vegetables, nuts and seeds, some fruit, plenty of healthy fats, very little starch, and zero dairy or sugar. Drink plenty of water and exercise consistently.

That is it.

Grains and legumes are not part of the diet.

Not much, huh?

Were you expecting some gimmick to set the diet apart?

Maybe a diet where you suck on a lemon before every meal. Or a diet where you avoid fat and eat only one solid meal per day. Or maybe a diet where you take enough herbal laxatives to poop out your spleen on the sidewalk.

Well, that is not happening here.

The Quantum Paleo program is about making a mental shift. When the mind shifts, losing weight becomes exponentially easier. When you shift your mind, you can accomplish extraordinary things with your body, your health, and almost any area of your life.

Today there are many clever diets on bookstore shelves. The wisdom in Quantum Paleo is so simple that you might overlook it.

The word diet comes from the Greek word *diaita*, which means "way of living."

During the first 21 days of the program you will tighten up what you eat. You will eat clean. You will eat at regular intervals. You will eat smaller portions.

There is nothing weird or extreme about it. Otherwise you would be setting yourself up for something you cannot maintain.

I am going to ask you to have one full day of eating healthy. Then the next day, do it again. Now repeat this discipline for 21 days in a row.

There are no gimmicks.

When the 21 days are complete, decide if you need to do another round. If you do, take three days off and start again. If you are happy with your body after one round, move on to Round 8 and read *Staying in the Pocket.*

Quantum Paleo breaks down like this:

Preparation

A. Deciding what you are fighting for
B. Getting your mind right

Taking Action

A. Doing the program
B. Performing one or more rounds (21-day units)

Staying in the Pocket

A. Stay on top
B. Maintain and improve

Stay Connected

A. Continue educating yourself about health
B. Join a community of people who stay fit

Question

Are you going to be like I was in India and watch from the sidelines?

This translates to buying this book, or reading it in the snack area of Barnes and Noble for an hour, then leaving it behind for someone else to put away because you decided the book is not for you.

Quit now. That is what my instructor said to me. Quit now. Or get in there and play as if your life depends on it.

I am telling you right now that Quantum Paleo is not the best diet ever written. There will always be someone who claims something else is better. The grass is always greener.

This program works because it is accessible and it gets to the core of how and why we change.

It will work for you too.

When you fight, compete, dance, or make love, there comes a moment when you have to stop thinking and analyzing. There comes a moment when you must stop being technical.

There comes a time to be fully present and simply do the task at hand.

Leap and the Net Will Appear!

This diet works if you do.

Are you ready to drink from the goblet?

Here it is …

Challenge #4

It's time to forgive yourself. Stop hating your past decisions. Let go of your regrets.

Forgiving yourself sets you free:

Free to lose weight.

Free to be happy.

Free to be in love again.

Free to be healthy.

Free to give your body exactly what it needs.

Free to transform your life.

Yes, you could bury this book in a time capsule and do ten more years of psychotherapy before attempting to get your body on track. That is one way.

Here is what I do with patients in my office. Purchase an ordinary notebook or journal.

Write at the top of the page:

"A list of all my regrets."

Start it this way:

A list of all my regrets (long list)

If I only …

If I would have …

If I could have …

If I finished …

If I never started …

For example:

"If I only took better care of my health."

"If I would have tried harder at my job."

"If I could have seen the economy declining sooner and made better adjustments."

"If I only finished high school."

"If I never started smoking cigarettes as a teenager."

Make your own list. It may be long. Keep going. Take as much time as you need. Add more regrets to the list.

Have the mindset of a cancer surgeon. Cancer surgeons know there is a significant risk if any of the bad tissue is left inside the body. You must cut it all out. Don't leave any of it behind. Get it all out. Write it down.

Now circle or place a check mark next to the worst ones. The regrets that feel like they have had the biggest impact on your life.

On a new sheet of paper, transfer the top five items you circled.

This becomes your new list:

Top 5 Regrets

At this point, you have a choice about how to handle this list. Both paths will work.

Here is the traditional way. Get counseling. Analyze it. Talk about it. Work on it for years if necessary. I am told that this works for some people.

It's not my way. I prefer that you do not do it this way.

Why?

Because I do not recommend spending enormous amounts of time on something that you will never be able to change.

Please understand that your "List of All My Regrets" and your "Top 5 Regrets" list is ancient history. The list only has power today if you constantly give it attention.

Let's say you regret not graduating from college. Because of this regret, you believe you are not making as much money as you could have.

What good does it do to keep replaying that today?

Nothing.

Does obsessing over your regrets get you a promotion or a college degree?

Does replaying it in your mind increase your income?

No.

What if your regret was that you wished you were closer with your mother before she died? Now she is gone and you cannot repair that relationship.

Here is something you can do.

Write her a long letter. Begin by explaining everything that you feel went wrong in the relationship. You get to go first. Tell her how she made you angry. If you felt she let you down, write it down. If you felt she was sometimes a lousy mother, say it.

Put it all down. Do not hold back.

Then tell her everything you love about her and everything you appreciate about her. Tell her how you could have been a better son or daughter. This is the time to be generous with praise, love, and compassion.

Close the letter with a paragraph explaining how you forgive her.

Then write a few sentences asking her to forgive you. Even if you believe it was mostly her fault. Ask anyway.

Be sincere in your forgiveness. Doing this kind of work can heal you at a deep level. This is the level where real transformation begins.

Obviously she will not be able to read this letter.

But you will.

Any relationship on your regrets list, whether the person is alive or not, can be improved in this way.

If the person is unreachable because they are dead, in prison, or unwilling to speak with you, write the letter anyway and keep it for yourself. This allows you to heal.

Make a decision to forgive yourself as well.

If the regret is financial, there may be nothing you can do about it. It happened. It hurts. But life is moving forward.

My wife and I were scammed several years ago. It wiped out nearly our entire nest egg. Trust me, it was significant. It reminded me of the Bernie Madoff scandal that everyone knows about. Eight years of saving money while working six days per week. Gone.

The people responsible went to jail. We never recovered our losses. Not only did we lose the money, but it damaged our taxes and credit score.

How painful is that? How embarrassing?

I cannot fully describe the pain it caused. It landed squarely on my Top 5 Regrets list. I was in a slump for almost a year afterward because we kept believing the situation might somehow be recovered.

It never was.

Not a penny came back.

Eventually I had to let it go. I refused to keep looking backward. We had to move on.

If the regret is related to health choices, such as:

"I wish I took better care of my body."

"I wish I started exercising when I was younger."

"I wish I never started smoking."

Then change it now.

Decide right this moment what you are fighting for and begin today.

It is over. Let it go.

From this day forward, improve every meaningful relationship in your life. It is worth it.

Did you know that when patients repair or end dysfunctional relationships, their health often improves rapidly? They lose weight. They sleep better. They feel inspired. They start exercising. They transform their lives.

People sometimes sign up just to lose ten pounds in three weeks and end up experiencing breakthroughs in entirely different areas of their lives.

Here is an optional closing ritual. My wife and I have done this together.

Write your Top 5 Regrets on a small piece of paper. Place it in a fire-safe container such as a fireplace. Say goodbye to the regrets. Kiss the paper. Then light it.

Yes, remember to kiss it before lighting it.

Watch it burn.

Then turn your back and walk away.

Never look back.

Back to the Kingdom of Success ...

Look down at the floor. There lies your cape of fear, regret, and self-loathing.

Step over the cape. Do not let it touch your feet.

Climb into the arena and prepare to fight.

Now I ask you again:

What are you fighting for?

Challenge #5

The 10 Questions You Must Answer

Below is a list of ten questions I often ask patients before they begin a new health journey. It is easy to skim past them, chuckle, and assume they do not apply to you.

But I feel strongly about these questions.

If you get clear about them, the diet becomes much easier.

Do you only want to lose ten pounds, or do you want to create breakthroughs in multiple areas of your life?

I want more for you than weight loss. I want you to take a quantum leap forward in many aspects of your life. I have seen it happen so often that I now expect it.

Here they are.

Get a pen and paper and write your answers. Get emotional about them. Daydream. Visualize. The more vividly you imagine these answers, the more real they will become.

1. What are you fighting for?
2. Who are you fighting for? (children, spouse, parents, etc.)
3. Other than yourself, whose life will be most affected when you transform your health and body?
4. What do you want to weigh, and by what date?
5. Example: 154 pounds by July 4th.
6. What area of your health needs the most improvement?

7. What disease or condition do you believe your body is most vulnerable to as you age?
8. For example: cancer, diabetes, heart disease, obesity.
9. What area of your fitness needs the most improvement?
10. Strength, endurance, flexibility, or conditioning.
11. What activities have you not been able to do recently?
12. Walking, running, climbing, traveling, dancing, lifting, etc.
13. Who might feel threatened or unhappy if you succeed?
14. There are sometimes people in our lives who are more comfortable when we fail.
15. What specific goals would you pursue if your health, energy, and body were at their best?
16. Career, paying off debt, education, relationships, hobbies, travel, learning a language, writing a book, running a marathon, climbing a mountain.

First write the questions in a notebook and answer each one honestly.

Then read them again and journal about how they make you feel. Write about the memories they trigger. Write about your dreams.

Keep your notebook private. Only share it with someone who has also completed their own list. No exceptions.

Only people who have done this exercise themselves will truly understand how to support you.

Blah, Blah, Blah

I am the king of excuses. How about you?

Excuses. Also known as could have, would have, should have.

Examples:

If my mother or father had only ______.

If my spouse had only ______.

If I had only finished that project.

If I had not spent time with those people.

If I had stayed on that path.

Listen, I do not hate your excuses.

I am too busy hating my own.

Actually, I hate yours too because they remind me of how much I hate mine.

Regrets can destroy a life. They fester. They rot your core. They corrode your spirit. They keep resurfacing like a monster in a horror movie.

They drain your energy and rob you of your future.

You might notice that I have strong feelings about this subject.

Here is another example.

"If I only did or didn't ______."

Come on. You have one too.

I have mine.

I graduated near the top of my high school class and went to Cornell University. Then I dropped out after three years. Twelve years later I finally finished my college degree.

It was not an Ivy League degree either.

I partied too much and wasted the opportunity. I regret that decision deeply.

I left school, moved to New York City, and did occasional acting work while also working as a waiter, bartender, and limousine driver.

I do not regret moving to New York or pursuing acting. I regret not finishing my degree at Cornell. That decision probably set me back ten years.

I was on a strong path and chose one that made my life far more difficult.

Yes, I have other regrets. We all do.

But I choose not to watch the reruns.

If I only...

It is possible to reinterpret the moments we regret and even forgive ourselves for them.

In my case, I now see leaving school as part of my life path. In a strange way, it may have been exactly where I was meant to go.

I eventually finished college and chiropractic school. All of the things I have done brought me here as the person I am today.

I am grateful for my wife, my children, and many things I might never have experienced had I taken another path.

But you know what?

Blah, blah, blah.

That is the sound your sad story makes in someone else's ears.

I am not talking about stories of hope or redemption. We love those stories. Everyone listens to stories of perseverance and triumph.

But stories about regret often sound like this:

Blah, blah, blah.

Here is a secret.

Most people do not want to hear a long list of your regrets. Not your spouse. Not your best friend. Not your mother. Especially not your children.

That is why therapists are paid to listen to those stories professionally.

Even when people politely listen, the background sound they hear is often: *blah, blah, blah.*

Even if I am wrong about that, ask yourself this question.

What good does repeating those regrets do for you?

Nothing.

Stop replaying them. They cost you too much.

Here is another insight.

Your regrets may be one of the reasons you are not losing weight.

They may be preventing you from getting healthy and moving forward with your life.

No regrets. Agreed?

Quantum Paleo begins in the next chapter.

This is the moment.

No one is forcing you to do this. No one can put cake in your mouth and sabotage your success. Only you can do that.

Are you already planning to fail?

Are you quietly preparing your excuses?

Or are you planning to win?

This is more than a diet. It is a tool that can become a catalyst for change in every area of your life.

How could that be?

Because this program requires you to take responsibility for your life.

If you let go of excuses and regrets, you can transform your body, your mind, and eventually many other areas of your life.

You will create momentum.

What if you are older, younger, or dealing with a physical limitation and it takes twelve rounds of 21 days to reach the level of health you want?

Then do twelve rounds.

What if you have no time, no money, and endless obstacles?

Blah, blah, blah.

Make it work. Or don't.

When I was 22 years old and living in Los Angeles, I had a friend named Catie who lived across the street.

One day we were talking about childhood and I made the mistake of complaining about my parents' divorce. I told her my entire "blah, blah, blah" story and explained how I believed I would be further along in life if those obstacles had not happened.

In other words, I was reciting my regret list.

Then it was her turn.

She told me about the day she found her father dead, hanging in their home when she was twelve years old. Six months later her mother committed suicide.

Catie and her four siblings were separated and sent to live with different relatives in different parts of the country. They barely saw each other again during childhood.

Catie is bright, funny, and incredibly creative. She never complained or made excuses.

If anyone could have justified living inside their regrets, it was Catie.

But she never did.

The truth is that everyone knows someone whose story is harder than their own.

Some people persevere against overwhelming odds. Others stagnate or collapse when difficulties arise.

We all have to choose.

There are a million reasons to fail at Quantum Paleo.

There are only two or three reasons you will succeed.

When you write down what you are fighting for, you will have all the reasons you need.

So I ask you again.

What are you fighting for?

Challenge #6

Write it down, now!

ROUND 5

TALE OF THE TAPE

The Wish List

When I teach a workshop I often ask a question that I first heard another speaker use years ago. I don't know who deserves credit for the idea. It may have been Brian Tracy or Jim Rohn.

First, I ask workshop participants to write down their goals. I notice that many people censor and filter their authentic dreams and desires. They may write something like:

I want to make 10 percent more income this year.

I want to cut my cigarettes down by three per day.

Or, I want to drop half a pound per week for the next four weeks.

Translation: I'm playing it safe.

Why?

Adults have lived long enough to be disappointed. We have had our bubble burst more than once.

We stopped believing in Santa Claus.

Have you ever seen a little kid sitting on Santa's lap? The child has zero filters. When Santa asks, "What do you want this Christmas?" the kid starts thinking big.

"I want a new house, a pony, a bicycle, a flat screen TV, and I want to go to Disney. I also want to grow six inches in the next two weeks and ..."

Does the kid say, "I want a pony, but only if my mutual fund performs better than it has in recent years?"

No. The child just says what he or she really wants.

Here is the big question. What would you ask for if you were a kid sitting on Santa's lap?

That's what I want to know.

Take out a piece of paper and write down how much weight you want to lose. Write the number down.

Who wrote the number? Was it the cautious adult part of you or the child inside of you?

I want the child to write the goal because adults often become too cautious or tentative.

Do you see how people hesitate to write down anything big? Small feels safe. Big feels scary.

Give the pen, or crayon, to the child inside of you and let that part answer these questions.

I asked many of these questions in the previous section. I am not having a senior moment. I want you to answer them again.

Take out a fresh page in your journal. This time think big. Let your uncensored mind pick up the crayon or pencil and write down your real goals.

Then you can compare them with what you wrote before. If you have not participated up to this point, that's okay. Pick up the pencil and start now. No regrets.

How much weight do you really want to lose?

How many 21-day rounds will it take?

How many times per week will you exercise?

What type of exercise will you do?

What other health goals do you have?

What internal systems in your body need improvement?

(Heart, lungs, immune system, etc.)

When was the last time you were truly happy with your weight?

What are you fighting for?

What is the second most important thing you are fighting for?

Who are you fighting for?

Anyone else?

What would change in your life if you met your goals?

How would you see yourself differently?

What would others think about your progress?

When was the last time you lived your life full out?

Do you plan on doing Quantum Paleo with a partner?

Do not skip this step or I will come to your house with a crayon and make you do it with me.

The late motivational speaker Jim Rohn said:

"The future does not get better by hope, it gets better by plan. And to plan for the future we need goals."

And this quote by W. W. Ziege:

"Nothing can stop the person with the right mental attitude from achieving his goal; nothing on earth can help the person with the wrong mental attitude."

Make your wish list now.

This is not a request.

The Only Diet That Counts

You must measure. We need to know our starting point. We need to know how much we weigh. We need to know our waist measurement, chest measurement, and hip measurement.

Buy a tape measure and measure around your belly button. Do it three times and calculate the average. Write it down. Do not let clothing interfere with the measurement.

Next measure your chest three times across the nipples with your arms relaxed at your sides. Record the average.

Next measure your hips around the widest part of your buttocks.

If possible, get someone to measure your body fat percentage. Write it down and date it. This information is helpful but not necessary to proceed.

Here are additional things you can measure if you choose. It can be motivating to see all the changes once you apply yourself.

If you decide to order blood work, ask your doctor to include the following tests:

Lipid profile

Hemoglobin A1c (to evaluate average blood sugar over the last three months)

Total cholesterol

Triglycerides

LDL

HDL

Fasting morning glucose

Request the full panel with Hemoglobin A1c included.

Daily Caloric Intake

Go to Google, and search for Daily Caloric Intake Calculator:

Enter your numbers into the Daily Caloric Intake calculator to estimate your calorie needs.

Then divide that number by five. That will be the approximate number of calories per meal.

For example, if the calculator estimates 2000 calories per day, divided by five meals that equals about 400 calories per meal.

Three scrambled eggs with mushrooms and one quarter of an avocado in an omelet, along with a double espresso, totals just under 400 calories.

If you are a smaller person, the numbers scale down. For example, if the calculator suggests 1200 calories per day, that could consist of three meals of 300 calories and two snacks of 150 calories.

Use the Daily Caloric Intake Calculator only as a starting place.

The next step is to track your calories for the first 21 days. At minimum track them for the first week. This will teach you where you stand.

Many mobile phones have calorie tracking apps. You can also use sites such as Livestrong.com for free tracking tools and MyFitnessPal.com

Keep in mind that these tools do not teach Paleo eating.

Counting and measuring is tedious but effective. Remember, this is not necessarily for the rest of your life. I recommend counting calories for at least seven days, preferably the full 21 days of the first round.

If you need to lose a significant amount of weight, I suggest tracking calories for six to twelve months or until you reach your goal.

Once you understand your numbers, we can make adjustments. For example, if you are not losing weight after five days, you may need to reduce your daily intake by 100 to 150 calories.

Are you exercising four or five times per week?

Are you sleeping as well as possible?

Are you drinking enough water?

To master your body and maximize results, write everything down.

If you had a coach, that person would track it for you. Become your own coach.

Knowing your numbers protects you from failure.

A Few More Things You Can Do

Keep a Journal

I have kept journals since I was 18 years old. I constantly write down thoughts, goals, plans, and dreams. I do not write every day, but year after year I fill journal after journal.

Some of my goals are so ambitious they might appear delusional if my journal ever fell into the wrong hands. I do not share my journals with anyone. They are private.

Keeping a journal helps you stay on track. You can record your measurements and your goals for safekeeping.

Take Before and After Photos

Take a photograph wearing shorts or a bathing suit with your arms relaxed at your sides. Take a front view, side view, and back view.

It is powerful to compare before and after photos when you reach your goals. Most phone cameras are sufficient for this task.

Document Your Success Story

Where did you start?

How long did it take?

What were your results?

What were you fighting for?

How did the transformation feel?

What changed in other areas of your life such as relationships, finances, creativity, or career?

Keep the essay between 500 and 700 words.

Share your story with a trusted friend or partner. You can also write a letter to your future self. Seal it in an envelope and open it one year from now.

When people choose to live out loud with their goals, they create powerful momentum.

To Weigh or Not to Weigh

That is the question.

Not for me. I strongly recommend weighing yourself every day.

During the Quantum Paleo program, weigh yourself every morning for 21 days. First thing when you wake up. Use the bathroom, remove clothing, then step on the scale.

Why?

Because we need data. The initial phase of this program lasts only 21 days.

I do not want to lose an entire week wondering whether you are on track. If you are not progressing after a few days, you must reevaluate calories, exercise frequency, or intensity.

Most diet programs recommend weighing yourself once per week because daily fluctuations can be discouraging. I take a different approach.

Weigh yourself every day. That is your homework.

There is power in knowing.

For example, I want you to notice if you retain water during certain phases of your menstrual cycle.

I want you to notice how your weight shifts before, during, or after menstruation.

I want you to see how sodium intake affects water retention.

I want you to observe how the scale reacts after four glasses of wine and a late night peanut butter and jelly sandwich.

I also want you to see how consistent diet and cardio sessions improve your numbers.

Daily weighing creates accountability.

If you have a 21 day deadline, measure every day.

Many programs advise weekly weighing. I understand that viewpoint, but I want people to learn to understand their bodies.

For example, someone might come to my office wanting to lose 75 pounds. That person may not have exercised in years. I want them to take a daily inventory.

I do not want them blindly following instructions. I want them actively learning about their body.

They weigh themselves daily, count calories for three weeks, track sleep, water intake, and digestion. As they gather this information, they begin to understand how their body responds.

Once people learn to understand their bodies, they gain the ability to control their weight and influence their health.

How often do we hear someone say, "I don't know what happened. I somehow gained 30 pounds over the last two years."

If the scale is not trending downward, adjustments must be made. Eat less, exercise more, or consult a physician if metabolic or hormonal issues may be involved.

Know your numbers. It is powerful.

Counting Calories

I hate counting calories. I do not recommend it.

Actually, sometimes I do.

When?

Let me explain. When it comes to diet coaching I typically see three types of clients.

Client Type 1

Age 25 to 45, generally in decent shape, but wants to lose 10 to 15 pounds. They were often athletic earlier in life and still exercise occasionally.

This person usually just needs education about food choices. They adopt a Paleo style of eating and maintain consistent workouts. Over several months they move toward their ideal body composition without much tracking.

Client Type 2

Any age, significantly overweight, and out of shape for many years. They may not remember the last time they were physically fit.

For this person I strongly recommend daily weighing for 21 days and calorie tracking for at least seven days, preferably the full 21 days.

Client Type 3

Someone who has experienced a major health scare and must radically change their eating habits. Their life and health depend on it.

In these cases I often use my 21 day Paleo Purification Program, which combines the Quantum Paleo diet with a detox protocol. After the cleanse they transition to Quantum Paleo as a lifestyle.

These clients track calories and weight daily for the first 21 days with strict adherence to the program. No grains, no legumes, no sugar, no alcohol, and no dairy.

Why?

Clients in categories 2 and 3 often lack the internal awareness that athletes or highly health conscious people develop over time.

Simply giving them the "perfect diet" is not enough. They must learn to understand how their body responds.

I want them eating healthy proteins, vegetables, fruits, seeds, nuts, and healthy fats while drinking water as their primary beverage. That is the Quantum Paleo framework.

But I also want them weighing daily, journaling about food, sleep, and digestion.

Counting calories for at least seven days, ideally 21 days, sometimes even six months to a year.

They must become responsible for their body.

Many people truly do not understand why their body gains or loses weight.

Track what goes in. Track what comes out. Learn the math.

Weight gain happens when calorie intake exceeds energy expenditure. Weight loss happens when intake falls below maintenance requirements.

Understanding your body's math is powerful.

Think about an attentive parent caring for a newborn. The parent notices everything. The baby's digestion, sleep patterns, skin, and behavior. They observe closely because they are responsible for the child's well being.

Who is paying that level of attention to your body?

Many adults have ignored their bodies for decades.

Sometimes experienced Paleo followers tell me they do not need calorie tracking.

If you are already nutrition savvy or highly athletic, you probably can skip this step.

But many of the people I work with need guidance.

Making a quantum shift in your relationship with food and health is far more important than simply losing weight.

Learn your numbers. Learn your patterns. Then make the changes that support your health and body composition.

ROUND 6

THE PRE-FIGHT

Sex and Wine

I decided to allow two glasses of wine per week on Quantum Paleo, but sex is unlimited.

Why?

Sex, for some people, is the only time they are not thinking about food.

When I was attending chiropractic school, I had a nutrition professor, Dr. T., who was disliked by the majority of students. I actually found Dr. T. inspiring. When it came to how people should eat, he was strict. A perfectionist. Unbendable.

Outside of teaching, he had a private practice in Atlanta, Georgia. He consulted with patients who were extremely ill. Using diet and nutrition alone, he was able to turn around many long-term chronic conditions.

My wife Rachel and I decided to take Rachel's mother, Trudy, to see Dr. T. Trudy was in decent health overall, but in her late seventies she was experiencing chronic arthritis pain in her knees, shoulders, and spine. She also had recurring upper respiratory infections every winter.

Dr. T. ordered several tests, including a food allergy test (ELISA IgG Food Assay). I still order this test for my patients in my office. After reviewing the results, he told Trudy to eliminate all grains, dairy, and sugar, along with another dozen minor foods that appeared on her blood test.

Trudy was a World War II concentration camp survivor. She had been brutalized, imprisoned, starved, and separated from her brother and mother, who were eventually executed at another camp.

Somehow she survived those years. She once told us that during her imprisonment she dreamed about the chance to eat a simple piece of bread and creamy brie. After the war she cherished a daily ritual of eating a baguette with a slice of brie every afternoon.

Now Dr. T. was demanding that she quit her bread and cheese.

Trudy did not want to see Dr. T. in the first place. Rachel and I had pushed her into the appointment. Trudy lasted about three minutes on that diet. She simply refused to follow his advice.

Here is my point.

When I sit down with a patient, I ask about their health and body goals. I try to find out what they are fighting for. Then I suggest small incremental steps that are reachable and attainable.

I learn what they currently eat and design a customized program that stays as close as possible to the foods they already enjoy. If someone has spent their life eating pizza, junk food, and low quality foods, I start by asking them to eat better meats and proteins. Then I encourage them to add vegetables. I also have them switch from soda and fruit juice to water as their primary beverage. High quality ingredients become the priority.

The 21-day diet is a short blast. During that time I will ask you to eliminate a few of your favorite foods.

In Round 8 of this book you will learn how to live with trade-offs. A trade-off means you keep one thing if you are willing to give up another. Exercise is another example. Some people exercise more frequently so they can occasionally enjoy certain foods while maintaining their ideal weight.

After reaching your ideal weight with Quantum Paleo, you might treat yourself to a glass or two of wine at a restaurant. For example, you might order a steak with a salad and vegetables while skipping the bread and dessert. That is the trade-off. Have the wine, skip the bread and dessert.

That is how you maintain your hard-won results.

Do you want to keep looking good naked or not?

If Trudy had been my patient, I would have kept her on the bread and brie.

Why?

For several reasons.

If I had conducted a proper interview, I would have discovered that bread and brie were the highlight of her day. She was 77 years old and determined to keep that ritual in her life until the day she died.

She was thin. She never overate. She swam five mornings a week. She had many positive habits already in place. The only prescription medication she was taking was for Type 2 diabetes.

My plan would have been to allow her bread and brie every afternoon as a starting point and design the rest of the day around it. She needed small meals every three hours. I was surprised that no one had previously educated her about diet and blood sugar management.

I would have recommended some supplements and increased her water intake. I also would have suggested eliminating all other dairy, grains, and sugar except for her daily bread and brie ritual.

Why keep dairy and grains if I criticize them elsewhere?

Because I am first a healthcare provider. I am not a Paleo evangelist. Trudy never expressed interest in a Paleo diet. Forcing Paleo on her caused her to quit within 24 hours.

Who wins in that scenario? Nobody.

My experience working with patients has taught me that it is better to meet people where they are and increase the level of change gradually.

If Trudy had been educated about the potential dangers of dairy and grains based on her test results, she could have recognized that bread and brie were her "cheat foods." As the rest of the diet improved, she could decide how often she wanted to indulge.

Many patients gain momentum once they begin feeling better. They gain energy, make better choices, and begin taking responsibility for their health.

Trudy might have succeeded with being off grains 95 percent of the day. We will never know. She continued eating bread and brie until the day she died in a car accident a few years later.

We love you, Oma.

Some patients are willing to radically change everything within seconds of my recommendations. Others require gradual progress. My job is to create a path for different personalities to succeed.

If Trudy had been suffering from inflammatory bowel disease or celiac disease, the conversation would have been very different. The more severe the illness, the more difficult the dietary choices may need to be.

Back to the wine.

Twenty-one days is a short period of time. Ideally you would complete Quantum Paleo with little or no wine. However, if wine were completely forbidden, many people would cheat.

About 50 percent of people can easily avoid wine for 21 days. About 10 percent do not drink at all. But the remaining group struggles.

So I decided to include two glasses of wine per week in the plan.

Two glasses per week. Not three. Not five. Zero is also allowed.

There is something valuable about learning moderation with two glasses rather than total abstinence. If I forced total abstinence, many people would spend the entire 21 days waiting for Day 22 so they could binge.

Have one glass midweek and one on the weekend, or both on the same night. Red or white wine is fine. No beer or hard liquor.

If you choose to drink wine, monitor your calories carefully that day. Add an extra cardio session during the week if necessary. You may also reduce portion sizes slightly. Each glass of wine contains roughly 150 to 190 calories.

Can you incorporate those calories into your daily total and still stay on track? That is the mindset required.

Build it into the plan.

Drinking every night will not work.

Dr. T.'s perfect diet may be ideal for very sick people, and I have used it successfully in severe cases. However, only a small percentage of people can follow a perfect diet indefinitely. One of my goals has been helping large numbers of people get results even if their willpower is imperfect.

After reaching your goal weight, the Post-Fight program described in Round 8 allows greater flexibility. It may include a small glass of wine with dinner on three nights per week, and two glasses on a fourth night.

First you must learn the balancing act.

If you are dealing with a serious illness, work one-on-one with a qualified nutrition professional. This book is designed for relatively healthy individuals who want to improve their vitality and regain control of their bodies.

My goal is to help you lose weight fast enough to stay motivated while still allowing occasional comfort foods to keep morale high. Over the last 14 years working with patients in New York City, I have simplified this program again and again.

Simple works.

Complicated plans belong to scholars and researchers.

Sex.

You can have as much sex as you want on this diet. It burns calories and generally improves your outlook on life.

And yes, I titled this section "Sex and Wine" because I knew it would get your attention.

What you should take away from this section is simple.

Do not aim for perfection. Aim for near-perfection in short 21-day bursts. Learn moderation and balance.

"Sex and wine" are really metaphors for life's pleasures and indulgences that challenge us to stay on track.

Make room for those moments and learn to manage them wisely.

Did You Go?

"Did you go?" my Grandma Irma would ask whenever I stayed at her house for the weekend. She was very concerned about my bowel movements.

The embarrassing part is that she was still asking me this question when I was fourteen years old. Sometimes in front of my friends. Eventually even in front of my first girlfriend.

Somehow that ritual skipped a generation with my mother. Now I have become the next Grandma Irma. I ask my patients the same question.

Question: How many bowel movements should you have per day?

Answer: At least one per day.

Many nutrition experts suggest that one bowel movement per meal is ideal. I will add that the stool should be well formed.

Some people never look. Take a look. It matters.

Dr. T., my nutrition professor, always said to work on the bowel first. No matter what disease or condition was present, he believed the digestive system had to function properly. Over the years I have found this to be sound advice.

I have interviewed many patients who believed having a bowel movement every two or three days was normal. Their doctor told them it was acceptable.

It may be common. It is not ideal.

Your stool is your body's waste. Remove the garbage. Do not allow it to accumulate. Proper elimination is a key pillar of health.

Quantum Paleo includes large amounts of fiber from vegetables and fruits, along with water and healthy fats. For many people this is sufficient. Others may benefit from supplements such as probiotics or fish oil.

As flour, dairy, and sugar are removed from the diet, bowel function often improves.

In my practice we also use an herbal formula that safely supports regular elimination.

The bottom line is simple.

You should be having a bowel movement every day.

Lose Weight Sleeping

Can you lose weight while sleeping?

Yes.

In December, I went away for five days during the holidays. Five days turned into ten because a blizzard cancelled our flight back to New York.

At first I was stressed because I had patients scheduled between Christmas and New Year's. After rescheduling appointments, I decided to enjoy the extra time in Florida with my family.

Enjoyment, for my family, usually involves food.

My wife and son are both classically trained chefs, so wherever we go food becomes the central event.

During those ten days I ate an enormous amount of food and drank plenty of wine. I assumed I had gained at least five to seven pounds. There was no scale where we were staying, so I could not check.

I exercised once during the entire trip.

When I finally returned to Brooklyn and stepped on the scale, I had lost one pound.

How could that happen?

The difference was sleep.

During my normal work schedule in New York I often go to bed around 11:30 p.m. and wake at 4:45 a.m., averaging about five and a half hours of sleep per night.

During those ten days in Florida I averaged about nine hours per night.

Why does this matter?

Cortisol.

Cortisol is a hormone produced by the adrenal glands. These glands influence almost every cell in the body. They are responsible for releasing hormones such as adrenaline, cortisol, aldosterone, and norepinephrine.

When we experience chronic stress, cortisol levels remain elevated. This promotes fat storage around the abdomen, hips, thighs, face, neck, and back.

High cortisol also disrupts sleep, creating a vicious cycle of fatigue, weight gain, and metabolic dysfunction.

Sleep deprivation affects the immune system, blood sugar regulation, memory, energy levels, and libido.

How much sleep is enough?

If you could sleep without an alarm clock for several days, how long would your body choose to sleep?

For most people, 7.5 to 8.5 hours per night appears to support optimal health and easier weight management.

If you have been functioning well on five to seven hours and rarely get sick, you may be an exception. But if you struggle with fatigue, weight gain, or frequent illness, improving sleep is one of the first things to address.

Sleep is one of the core pillars of health alongside food, air, and water.

If you are tired all the time, start by evaluating your sleep.

Before changing anything, run a simple experiment. For five nights record the time you go to bed, the time you wake up, and rate the quality of your sleep on a scale from 1 to 10.

Then improve your sleep environment. Darken the room completely, remove unnecessary electronics, adjust the temperature, and go to bed earlier. Track the next five nights and compare the results.

Better sleep improves mental clarity, immune function, libido, and weight management.

It is one of the most powerful tools you have.

Exercise or Die

Pretty strong statement.

It holds a lot of truth.

Maybe a more palatable statement would be this: exercise if you want some influence over how you age and how you die. Or perhaps exercise can change the way you die. As my daughter might say, "I'm being a little dramatic."

Maybe we can settle on this: exercise can change the way we live. Yes, that is better.

I really enjoyed the book *The Paleo Solution* by Robb Wolf. He is a research biochemist, athlete, and coach who wrote an excellent book on the Paleolithic diet. He is considered one of the leading voices in Paleolithic nutrition. He writes and lectures about diet, exercise, hormone balance, and how we genetically resemble our hunter-gatherer ancestors from the Paleolithic era.

He outlines how we should eat and live to get as close as possible to our genetic potential for health and fitness. Chapter nine focuses on the importance of exercise and how it relates to genetic expression.

Do not let the phrase genetic expression scare you off. Wolf has a way of making dense material funny, engaging, and easy to understand.

He writes on page 146:

"Our hunter-gatherer ancestors lived an active, vigorous life. They and their prehuman ancestors had to expend remarkable amounts of energy to provide food, clothing, and shelter. Over millions of years our genetics were forged with a level of activity not dissimilar from that of an Olympic caliber athlete. This is what our genetics expect when we are born into the world. We are literally born to be fit. An unfortunate side effect of technology and affluence is that the physical activity that made our ancestors strong and healthy is all but missing from our sedentary lives. On a molecular level this lack of exercise literally changes who we are."

Let me give you a quick summary of his main point.

Your genotype is the genetic blueprint you inherit from your parents. For example, imagine both of your parents were elite athletes. You might inherit some remarkable athletic potential.

But potential alone does not guarantee anything.

You could still live a sedentary life and never express that potential.

That expression of your genes is called your phenotype. As Wolf writes, how your genes experience the world through food, sleep, community, and exercise determines which genes are turned on or off. That determines your phenotype.

The image that comes to mind for me is the dimmer switch in your dining room. Assuming you have a dining room. Many of us in New York City have turned our dining rooms into extra bedrooms.

Your lifestyle controls that dimmer switch.

If you eat well, exercise, sleep properly, and build strong social connections, you can turn that dimmer switch toward your full genetic potential. If you live sedentary, stressed, and poorly nourished, you dim that switch down.

Imagine you have done very little exercise over the past year. A scientist could analyze your genetic activity during this sedentary state and estimate your future disease risk if nothing changes.

Now imagine you transform your lifestyle over the next six to twelve months. You exercise regularly, lose excess weight, sleep better, and eat the way your body was designed to eat.

If that same scientist analyzed your genes again, the pattern would look completely different.

You would have changed your phenotype.

The list of potential diseases might not resemble the earlier version of you at all.

So yes, exercise matters.

I often hear patients say, "I don't have time to exercise," or "I don't like exercise."

What I have learned over the years is that exercise is not optional. It belongs in the same category as food and air.

Imagine saying, "I don't have time for air," or "I don't enjoy breathing."

The *Journal of the American Medical Association* reported that poor diet and physical inactivity are among the leading causes of preventable death in the United States. One analysis estimated that roughly 400,000 deaths per year were associated with poor diet and inactivity.

That is more than 1,000 people per day.

To put that in perspective, imagine if three jumbo jets carrying 300 passengers crashed every day for an entire year. It would be the biggest news story of the century.

Yet when people die slowly because of lifestyle disease, it rarely gets the same attention.

The report concluded with this warning: smoking remained the leading cause of preventable death, but poor diet and inactivity were rapidly catching up.

On Quantum Paleo I want you to exercise four to five days per week.

Remember, the first phase is a sprint. Twenty-one days. Fifteen workouts.

At least three workouts should include thirty minutes or more of aerobic activity. If you are walking, the pace should make you slightly breathless.

If you are more advanced, push yourself a little harder.

From the first day the finish line is already in sight.

Get Fat

This section could easily become an entire book on its own. At the back of this book I recommend several excellent books that explore the science in much greater depth.

I want this book to focus more on the mindset and the practical steps rather than heavy science.

In Robb Wolf's book *The Paleo Solution*, he makes an important point about cardiovascular disease and saturated fats.

He writes that a high intake of saturated fat combined with a high intake of carbohydrates can be a dangerous combination. However, when carbohydrate intake is moderated and fats come from natural sources, the risk picture changes dramatically.

The key point is simple.

There are good fats and bad fats.

Healthy fats include those from grass-fed meats, wild-caught fish, olive oil, coconut oil, avocados, olives, seeds, and nuts.

Highly processed vegetable oils such as corn oil, soy oil, and safflower oil tend to be overly rich in certain inflammatory fatty acids and should be minimized.

Artificial trans fats, such as those once common in margarine and processed foods, should be avoided entirely.

Keep it simple. Focus on whole foods and natural sources of fat.

If you want to explore the deeper research on this subject, I recommend authors such as Robb Wolf, Loren Cordain, Gary Taubes, Mark Sisson, and Nora Gedgaudas. Their books include extensive references to peer-reviewed research.

How Much Water?

It depends. Everyone is different.

Most people are not drinking enough water.

Water that appears in coffee, tea, or soft drinks technically counts, but it is not an ideal source. I once had a patient who told me she never drank water. When I asked about it, she corrected herself and said she did have a splash of water with her scotch.

There are different guidelines. One common suggestion is to drink half your body weight in ounces per day. If you weigh 200 pounds, that would equal about 100 ounces of water daily.

Another popular guideline is the classic eight glasses per day rule.

I tend to suggest the body weight guideline because it adjusts to the size of the individual. Age, activity level, climate, and overall health all influence hydration needs.

The average person also obtains roughly 20 percent of their daily water from food, particularly fruits and vegetables.

Over the years I have noticed two general types of patients.

The first group is healthy and athletic. They seem to intuitively know how much sleep, water, and exercise they need.

The second group struggles more with building health and needs clearer guidelines.

If that sounds like you, start by drinking at least two liters of water per day for one week. After that, experiment with the half body weight guideline and see how your body responds.

We are all biochemically unique. Water intake should be adjusted based on how you feel and perform.

Twenty-One Days

Why twenty-one days?

I used to challenge patients with ninety day programs. At one point I even ran six month programs.

Most people struggle to commit to anything for six months.

Think about how hard it is to schedule your next dental cleaning six months in advance.

Twenty-one days feels manageable.

It is short enough to stay motivated, but long enough to see real change. You can almost see the finish line from the starting line.

Give me twenty-one days.

That is what I ask.

If you need more time after that, you can repeat the cycle. But first focus only on the next twenty-one days.

Mark the start and finish dates on your calendar. I should be able to call you and ask, "What day are you on?" and you immediately know whether it is Day 11 or Day 17.

During those twenty-one days aim for four workouts per week. Five is even better.

That means at least twelve workouts. Possibly fifteen.

Small steps add up.

Most people cannot drop down and do fifty pushups. But many people can do ten, rest, then do another ten. Break the challenge into smaller pieces and suddenly it becomes possible.

Weight loss works the same way.

Small steps create momentum.

Over time those small steps can transform your life.

There is an old saying that it takes one month to repair your health for every year you have been off track.

Is that formula perfect? Of course not.

But it contains a useful truth. Transformation takes time.

This book is about rebuilding your health. Losing weight will not solve every problem, but it dramatically improves many aspects of health.

Decide to change.

Figure out why.

What are you fighting for?

Then start.

Do not worry about five years or even five months. Focus on the first twenty-one days.

How Much Weight Can You Lose in 21 Days?

I do not know.

Bryan L. lost twenty-six pounds in twenty-one days during a Quantum Paleo competition I ran in New York City in 2011.

Another participant lost 21.9 pounds and another lost 14.9 pounds.

Group settings can be powerful. Friendly competition often amplifies results. You might consider forming a small group at work, among friends, or within your family and running a twenty-one day challenge together.

You can repeat the rounds as many times as needed. Take a short break between rounds and begin again.

Even large goals such as losing 100 pounds become achievable when broken into smaller segments.

Round 7

The Fight Plan

"That's it?"

Maybe I should have named this section "That's It!"

When I explain the diet to people, they almost always ask the same question:

"Is that it?"

Yes. That is it.

The instructions are simple. Eat the foods you should eat and avoid the foods you shouldn't.

Why?

The recommended foods have been available to humans for more than two million years. During that time our bodies adapted to eating, digesting, and utilizing these types of foods.

Only in the last ten thousand years did humans begin regularly eating grains, beans, sugar, and milk from domesticated animals. From an evolutionary perspective, that is a very short period of time.

These foods are relatively new additions to the human diet, and not everyone digests them well. Many people experience health problems when grains, sugar, dairy, and legumes become major staples of their daily diet.

Think about it this way.

What would happen if you fed your family dog nothing but fast food, pizza, beer, ice cream, bagels, pancakes, potato chips, and peanut butter sandwiches? Would you expect that dog to be healthy?

Actually, that may not be the best example. Dogs have been domesticated for thousands of years and many already eat processed foods from cans or bags. Some people already feed their dogs foods like this.

A better example would be taking a wild animal that eats its natural diet and forcing it to eat foods that are completely foreign to its biology. That experiment would almost certainly result in poor health.

Poor nutrition can even affect future generations. (Pottenger, Francis M. *Pottenger's Cats: A Study in Nutrition.*)

The Diet

It is not complicated.

Here it is.

The diet consists of proteins, vegetables, nuts and seeds, some fruit, plenty of healthy fats, very little starch, no dairy, and zero sugar.

That is it.

Grains and legumes are not included in the diet.

Let's Walk Through One Day

Wake up.

Meal 1 (8:00 a.m.)

Protein, fat, coffee or tea, and fruit.

Example: a two-egg omelet with mushrooms, onions, avocado, and diced turkey sausage. Espresso or tea. A sliced apple on the side.

Meal 2 (12:00 p.m.)

Protein, vegetables, salad.

Example: a salad with grilled chicken, olive oil and vinegar, and olives.

Meal 3 (4:00 p.m.)

Snack.

Example: celery or carrot sticks with one to two tablespoons of almond butter.

Or a hard-boiled egg and a small apple.

Meal 4 (7:30 p.m.)

Protein, vegetables, fat, and a little starch.

Example: grilled chicken, fish, or meat with vegetables and salad with oil and vinegar, plus half a yam.

Optional Snack Times

Mid-morning

Some people do very well with a mid-morning snack.

Example: leftover protein from dinner with a small slice of avocado.

Or 10 to 12 raw almonds and carrot sticks.

Late night

If you are still awake four hours after dinner, have another small healthy snack.

That's it.

Adding Variety

How do you keep it interesting?

There are many excellent Paleo cookbooks available. I list several in the Resources section of this book.

Calorie Awareness

If you are serious about losing weight, I recommend getting a reasonable estimate of your daily calorie intake.

In Round 4, "Tale of the Tape," I discussed tracking your calories for at least one week, ideally the full 21 days.

Tracking calories gives you awareness. It does not have to become a lifelong habit, but during the initial phase it can be extremely helpful.

Everyone's metabolism is different, so these numbers are only starting points. You may need to adjust them based on your progress.

Example: 1300 Calorie Plan

Meal 1

Protein + fruit

One egg with an apple, orange, pear, or berries. Coffee or tea.

Calories: about 220

Meal 2

Protein + vegetables

Small salad with chicken or salmon plus vegetables. Olive oil and vinegar. Avocado or olives.

No bread, croutons, or cheese.

Calories: about 350

Meal 3

Snack

Examples:

One hard-boiled egg with carrots

or

one tablespoon almond butter with celery or carrot sticks

or

sliced turkey with a quarter avocado

or

eleven cashews and an apple

Calories: about 210

Meal 4

Protein + vegetables

About four ounces of meat, fish, or chicken with vegetables.

Calories: about 300

Meal 5

Optional snack

Two hard-boiled eggs.

Calories: about 140

Total: about 1220 calories

Example: 1900 Calorie Plan

Meal 1

Three eggs with fruit. Coffee or tea.

Calories: about 400

Meal 2

Salad with chicken or salmon, vegetables, olive oil and vinegar, avocado or olives.

Calories: about 400

Meal 3

Snack.

Examples:

two hard-boiled eggs with carrots

almond butter with celery or carrots

¼ pound sliced turkey with avocado

Fifteen cashews and an apple

Calories: about 300

Meal 4

Six ounces of meat, fish, or chicken with vegetables.

Calories: about 400

Meal 5

Optional snack.

Calories: about 300

Total: about 1800 calories

Summary

Calorie tracking is mainly useful for people who have a significant weight loss goal.

If your goal is maintenance or gradual improvement in body composition, you may not need to track calories at all.

But if you want faster results during the initial 21 days, weighing yourself and tracking your intake can be very helpful.

For example, if your daily calorie target is 1500 calories and you eat four meals per day, that means about 375 calories per meal.

If you eat five meals per day, that means about 300 calories per meal.

It is simple math.

Once you do the calculations once, the routine becomes easy. Repeat it for 21 days.

Taking responsibility for your numbers helps you master your body.

Tracking Tools

Many people use a free tracking tool such as **MyFitnessPal.**

It is usually easier to create your profile on a computer first, then use the mobile app to track meals throughout the day.

The app allows you to see how many calories you have left to eat at any given point.

You do not have to use a tracking app forever.

Use it long enough to learn the patterns of your eating and to prevent self-sabotage.

Once you understand your habits and portions, you may not need it anymore.

Flying By the Seat of Your Pantry

If you want to win this fight, your kitchen has to support you.

Most people fail diets not because they lack discipline, but because the wrong foods are the easiest foods to grab. When your pantry and refrigerator are filled with the right ingredients, good choices become automatic. When they are filled with junk, you will eventually eat junk.

Think of your kitchen as your training camp.

Stock it correctly and the rest of the program becomes much easier.

Cooking for yourself at home is valuable on many levels. For our purposes, it is especially helpful because it allows you to control what you eat, the quality of the ingredients, and how the food is prepared. When you cook at home, you rely less on take-out and processed foods that often contain hidden calories, grains, sugar, chemicals, artificial coloring, additives, and excessive sodium.

Here are some key ingredients and pantry items you may want to keep on hand so you can quickly prepare simple meals and recipes similar to those found in many Paleo cookbooks (see the Resources section for suggestions).

Herbs

Fresh herbs can stay fresh for up to a week if wrapped loosely in a damp paper towel and stored in an airtight bag or container. This works especially well for delicate herbs like cilantro, basil, and tarragon.

Another method for sturdier herbs is to treat them like flowers. Place them in a small container of water and store them in the refrigerator. This keeps them accessible and adds a bright splash of green every time you open the fridge.

Spices

Basic spices to keep on hand include cumin, garlic powder, onion powder, cayenne, red pepper flakes, curry powder, chile powder, dried thyme, dried oregano, coriander, Chinese five spice, ras el hanout, cinnamon, allspice, cloves, vanilla extract, smoked paprika, sweet paprika, cardamom, mustard powder, and black pepper.

Hot sauces such as Tabasco or Sriracha can also be useful.

Yes, whole spices ground fresh provide the most flavor. If you have the time and equipment, that is ideal. But pre-ground spices are perfectly fine. Just buy smaller quantities and replace spices that have been sitting in your pantry longer than six months. A simple trick is to write the purchase date on the jar with a marker.

Fats and Oils

Low-fat diets have become about as outdated as the advertisements that once suggested cigarettes were good for digestion.

Our bodies need fat. Fat improves flavor, texture, and satiety. Eating quality fat helps you stay full and satisfied.

However, not all fats are equal.

High-quality oils made from nuts such as almond, hazelnut, walnut, and macadamia, along with avocado oil and premium extra-virgin olive oil, are best used for finishing dishes or salad dressings rather than cooking.

For medium-heat cooking, less expensive olive oil works well. For high-heat cooking, coconut oil, clarified butter (ghee), or unprocessed palm oil are good options.

Note: delicate oils such as nut oils should be stored in the refrigerator. If they solidify, simply run the bottle under warm water before using.

Avoid canola oil, safflower oil, sunflower oil, soybean oil, grapeseed oil, cottonseed oil, margarine, and other hydrogenated oils.

Clarified butter (ghee) can also be used for cooking.

Nuts and Seeds

Nuts and seeds make excellent snacks. They provide healthy fats and the satisfying crunch many people miss when they remove grains from their diet.

Moderation is important. A small amount goes a long way.

Ideally buy raw nuts and seeds and lightly roast them in your oven at about 300 degrees for 8–12 minutes if you prefer them roasted.

They can be chopped, grated, or ground into recipes to add flavor and texture to salads, dressings, sautéed vegetables, fruit dishes, or smoothies.

Refrigeration helps maintain freshness.

Broths

Vegetable, chicken, and beef broths are widely available in grocery stores. However, unless you can find versions labeled organic, low sodium, and MSG-free, you may be better off making your own.

Homemade broth can be frozen in small containers and used later to make soups, sauté vegetables, poach proteins, or add flavor to many dishes.

Non-Dairy Milks

Many non-dairy milks can be surprisingly high in sugar or carbohydrates. Choose unsweetened varieties.

Avoid soy milk. Better alternatives include almond, coconut, or hemp milk.

Coconut milk in cans works well for cooking. Carton versions from the refrigerated section are often used in smoothies or coffee.

Always avoid products with added sweeteners or high-fructose corn syrup.

Flour Alternatives

Coconut flour and nut flours are useful alternatives. Because nuts contain oils that can spoil, buy smaller quantities and store them in the refrigerator.

Sweeteners

Avoid artificial sweeteners whenever possible. Even "natural" sugar substitutes can keep your brain craving sweetness.

If a recipe truly requires sweetener, use moderate amounts of maple syrup, raw honey, or minimally processed sugar instead of artificial substitutes.

Cheese, Yogurt, and Dairy

During the first 21 days you should avoid dairy completely.

After that period you may reintroduce it carefully if desired. Dairy is calorie dense and often produces excess mucus for some people.

If you choose to eat dairy, moderate amounts of aged cheeses or goat and sheep milk cheeses may be better tolerated than heavily processed cheeses made from cow's milk.

Plain unsweetened yogurt can provide probiotic support and can be combined with fruit, nuts, seeds, or coconut.

However, some people simply do better without dairy. If you suspect dairy sensitivity, eliminating it entirely may be helpful.

My general recommendation is simple: no milk, cheese, or yogurt for the first 21 days. Give your body a break. After that you can experiment and determine how well you tolerate dairy.

Canned and Jarred Goods

These items can be helpful in a pinch.

Artichoke hearts

Hearts of palm

Tuna (low sodium)

Salmon

Sardines

Anchovies

Smoked oysters

Nut butters without added sugar or trans fats

Plum tomatoes

Salsa

Tapenades

Olives

Roasted peppers

Capers

Canned fruit packed in natural juice

Unsweetened applesauce

Unsweetened dried fruits such as apricots, raisins, or cranberries (in moderation)

Yams or sweet potatoes not packed in syrup

Most vegetables are better fresh or frozen rather than canned because canned vegetables often contain excess sodium and preservatives.

A Word on Buying Meats and Fish

The Quantum Paleo lifestyle includes more meat, fish, eggs, and poultry than many modern diets, so quality matters.

Organic meat can be expensive and sometimes difficult to find, but availability continues to improve as consumer demand grows.

Farmers markets are often a good place to find high-quality meat and poultry.

If organic meat is not available or affordable, look for labels such as hormone-free, antibiotic-free, cage-free, or grass-fed.

Wild-caught seafood is generally preferable when possible.

The Monterey Bay Aquarium Seafood Watch program offers guidance on seafood that is considered safe and sustainable. You can search for it as ISEAL

Planning and Preparation Give You the Edge in This Fight

Quantum Paleo allows you to eat plenty of food. You will not starve.

The key to success is feeding your body foods that maximize energy, vitality, and balanced calorie intake. This requires some planning, but it is not complicated.

You will be eating four to five times per day. Packing snacks or lunch for work or travel helps prevent the moment when hunger takes over and you grab whatever food is available.

If you spend a few hours on a weekend preparing a few staple foods, you can quickly assemble healthy meals during the week.

Examples include:

Hard-boil two dozen eggs and store them in an airtight container.

Grilled or baked chicken breasts or thighs.

Roasted tomatoes or peppers.

Roasted root vegetables.

Blanched vegetables such as broccoli or asparagus.

Roasted nuts.

Always Have on Hand

Baby carrots

Apples, pears, or other fruit you enjoy

Celery and salad greens

Eggs

Sliced turkey, ham, or other meats (for roll-ups, salads, or quick protein additions)

Hunt and Gather Guide

For making choices on the fly, here is your basic list of YES foods and NO foods.

Yes Foods

Eggs

Nuts

Seeds

Coconut in all forms

Coffee and tea

Protein powders (avoid soy)

Beef, pork, poultry, and game meats

Grass-fed meat when possible

Wild-caught seafood

Fruits and vegetables

Salad greens

Healthy oils, vinegars, and lemon juice

No Foods

Whole grains and flour products

Bread, pasta, cake, bagels, cereals, and breaded foods

Beans and legumes

Artificial sweeteners

Fruit juice as a beverage

Sugar

Dairy during the first 21 days

Occasionally

Dark chocolate (60% cacao or higher)

Red wine

Cheese in moderation after the initial 21 days

Yams and sweet potatoes

Potatoes

A Word About Meal Labels and Habits

We live with labels such as "Breakfast," "Lunch," "Dinner," and "Snack." Each one immediately brings to mind a list of foods that seem appropriate for that meal.

Do you have fixed ideas about what a normal breakfast, lunch, dinner, or snack should look like? Are there meal combinations that you feel stuck with?

The typical American diet often looks like this: eggs, bread, smoked meats, cereal, pastries, and fruit for breakfast; sandwiches, burgers, fries, and salads for lunch; and a large meat, potatoes, vegetables, and dessert for dinner. Snacks often mean chips, pretzels, or candy bars that come from a bag or wrapper.

The Quantum Paleo lifestyle asks you to step outside those assumptions and become more flexible with how you think about meals. It encourages you to retrain your daily eating habits.

I often hear people box themselves into high-calorie habits with statements like these:

"I can't eat eggs without bread."

"I need something sweet for breakfast."

"A meal isn't complete without a starch."

"I'm a meat-and-potatoes person when it comes to dinner."

"I can't live without pasta a few times a week."

"I can't stand water. I need something sweet with my meals."

Try mixing things up.

Eat hard-boiled eggs as a snack instead of only at breakfast. Eat leftovers from last night's dinner for breakfast. A bowl of fruit with yogurt and nuts can be dinner. Finish dinner with a piece of cheese and an apple instead of a sugary dessert once you have completed the initial 21 days.

Make a small salad with nuts and unsweetened dried fruit for a mid-morning snack and you will avoid the sugar spike and crash that comes from candy bars or high-carb chips.

Being a Victor, Not a Victim

Quantum Paleo is an eating plan, but it is more than that. You will not succeed unless you become clear about what you are fighting for and decide that you are willing to fight for it.

Whatever your reason is, it must be strong enough to help you overcome habits, excuses, temptations, and the status quo of the modern diet.

Reaching your weight and health goals means choosing to become a victor over those challenges.

A victor thinks this way:

"I eat foods that contribute to my goals."

"I avoid foods that I know undermine my health."

"I make choices that support my well-being."

"I am in charge. If I eat something off plan, I return to the plan with the next meal."

"I deserve great health, a strong body, vitality, energy, and a clear mind."

"I accept healthy eating as a powerful lifestyle that puts me in control."

"I enjoy high-quality foods and take responsibility for my health."

You give away your power and move into a victim mindset when you say things like:

"I can't avoid cake or candy because my office always has treats."

"My work schedule doesn't allow me to eat healthy."

"I don't have time to eat well. I'm always on the go."

"I would eat better if my kids or spouse didn't keep junk food in the house."

"Someday, when the timing is right, I'll start eating better."

P.S. on Dairy

After the initial 21-day phase is complete, you will need to decide where you stand with dairy.

If you eliminated milk, cheese, and yogurt during the program, you may notice a reaction when you reintroduce them. Possible reactions include intestinal gas, bloating, stomach discomfort, excess mucus in the throat or sinuses, or changes in stool.

If you experience these reactions, dairy may be problematic for you.

Another option is to use a food sensitivity test to assess how your body responds to dairy and other foods.

These tests can evaluate your response to dairy, eggs, grains, and many other foods.

There are generally three categories of people when it comes to dairy:

Those who can eat dairy without any noticeable issues.

Those who cannot tolerate dairy at all.

Those who can tolerate certain types or amounts of dairy but not others.

It may take some experimentation to determine where you fall. Trial and error, observation, and occasionally testing can help clarify your personal tolerance.

In my experience, fewer than 40 percent of people have absolutely no issues with dairy.

Are you one of them?

ROUND 8

THE POST-FIGHT

Staying in the Pocket

Getting in the pocket. The zone. The groove. Hitting the sweet spot.

I use these phrases to describe when someone is in their optimal state of health. Everything in the body is working well, and the person's health feels predictable and consistent.

My practice tends to attract people who want to get into the pocket. I am not a medical doctor. I do not specialize in diagnosing or managing medical crises. What I focus on is helping people rebuild their health and move toward a stable, vibrant baseline.

First, I listen to their story. How did they arrive at their current situation? That story usually reveals important clues.

From there, I look for practical ways to help them rebuild their health. I examine diet, lifestyle, emotional balance, sleep, exercise, and the other fundamentals that influence well-being.

This process is similar to working with a personal trainer whose goal is to help you get physically fit.

My approach focuses on building health rather than chasing symptoms.

"As you build health, you become less sick."

"Sickness struggles to exist when you are living in the pocket."

Traditional disease management often focuses on identifying a malfunctioning system or organ and then prescribing medications to manage symptoms. Many medications are designed primarily to control symptoms rather than resolve the deeper causes of illness.

That does not mean medications are never necessary. But if someone wants to truly transform their health, they often need to take the longer path of rebuilding the body from the ground up.

Because I do not prescribe medications, it forces me to think differently.

"How can I strengthen this person's overall health?"

"What one or two changes might improve the entire system?"

This mindset pushes me to search for root causes and rebuild health from the foundation upward.

You might think this approach sounds overly simple.

It is not.

I would estimate that a large percentage of health problems develop gradually from lifestyle patterns. Diet, stress, inactivity, and environmental exposures all play a role. Of course, there are exceptions. Some diseases occur for reasons outside anyone's control.

But when you look at the leading causes of death in the United States, many of them are strongly influenced by lifestyle.

Leading causes of death in the United States have historically included heart disease, cancer, stroke, chronic respiratory disease, accidents, Alzheimer's disease, diabetes, influenza and pneumonia, kidney disease, and septicemia.

Heart disease, which consistently ranks near the top of the list, is strongly influenced by diet, exercise, and lifestyle habits.

Cancer can arise from many causes. Sometimes the reasons are unclear. In other cases environmental exposures, toxins, smoking, or chronic lifestyle stressors may contribute.

Modern life exposes us to chemicals, pollutants, and highly processed foods. Many crops are treated with pesticides. Food processing methods may include chemical preservatives or other additives designed to extend shelf life.

This reality makes food quality more important than ever.

That is why I encourage people to choose foods that are as natural and minimally processed as possible. Whenever you can, choose clean sources of meat, fish, vegetables, and whole foods.

Can better food, fewer processed ingredients, regular exercise, and reduced toxin exposure improve health?

Of course they can.

In my experience, when people adopt a structured eating plan such as the 21-day Quantum Paleo reset, their health often improves rapidly. Energy increases. Digestion improves. Sleep stabilizes. Lab markers sometimes improve as well.

When someone gets back into their pocket, many aspects of health begin moving in the right direction.

Energy improves. Libido improves. The immune system becomes stronger. Hormonal balance, digestion, sleep, skin quality, and mental clarity often improve as well.

One of my teachers once shared a simple guideline. For every year you have been out of balance with your health, it may take roughly a month of focused effort to restore it.

Is that formula perfect? Of course not.

But it reminds us that rebuilding health takes time and consistency.

Some people accelerate their progress when they commit fully to lifestyle changes. Others move more gradually. Either way, progress is possible.

Even people living with chronic conditions can often improve their vitality and quality of life significantly.

That alone is a goal worth fighting for.

The Ninja Mind Keeps the Weight Off

Maintaining weight loss requires a particular mindset.

Most people are not born with it. It has to be practiced.

For me, it has been a lifelong challenge. I am both the teacher and the student in this process.

My stepfather George is a master of self-control when it comes to food. He has a simple rule: "The mouth is in lockdown at 8 p.m."

When he decides he is done eating, that is it. No exceptions.

Chocolate does not tempt him. Wine does not tempt him. Nothing does.

For most of my life I was not wired that way. A little persuasion and I could easily be convinced to eat dessert or have a beer.

That was the old version of me.

The newer version of me practices what I call the Ninja Mind.

Some people use practical tricks. A friend of mine pours water over the remaining food on his plate once he decides he is finished. Others ask the waiter to remove their plate as soon as they feel satisfied. Some people brush their teeth immediately after dinner to signal that eating is finished.

Those strategies can help, but my real advice focuses on mindset rather than tricks.

The big question is this:

How do you bridge the gap between discipline and temptation?

I wish I could claim to have mastered this completely. I have not.

Even today, I still face the internal struggle between staying on plan and wanting something indulgent.

One afternoon I walked into a small café near my office. They had excellent coffee and a large chocolate sandwich cookie with cream filling.

Years ago my routine was simple: every afternoon I ordered coffee and that cookie.

Now I try to stay on track.

I stepped up to the counter and ordered a small coffee.

The person behind the counter recognized me.

"Would you like the double cookie today?"

In that moment my mind began spinning through options like a game show wheel.

Coffee and cookie.

Coffee only.

Maybe just one bite.

Maybe a different dessert.

On that imaginary wheel I could see images of cookies, ice cream, pizza, and other indulgences.

But I could also see two other images.

The unhealthy version of myself.

And the healthier version.

I grabbed the wheel and forced it to stop on coffee.

"No thank you."

The temptation did not disappear. The struggle was still real.

The difference was that my motivation had become stronger.

Today my "what are you fighting for?" is clear.

Two things drive me most strongly: my health and the desire to look and feel my best.

That commitment is bigger than my craving for a cookie or a slice of pizza.

Motivational speaker Tony Robbins once framed it this way: we must decide which pain is greater.

The pain of resisting short-term pleasure.

Or the pain of not achieving our long-term goals.

For many years I chose the short-term reward.

Now I try to choose the long-term outcome.

When your "what are you fighting for?" is clear and meaningful, it becomes easier to make better decisions.

There is no magic trick that eliminates temptation completely.

There are no gimmicks that permanently replace discipline.

Some people try to solve the problem with drugs or stimulants, but those shortcuts often create new problems.

The better path is simpler.

Decide what you are fighting for.

Commit to the first 21 days.

Eat smaller meals four to five times per day.

Exercise consistently.

Practice making decisions that support your long-term health.

When the first 21 days are complete, take a short break and repeat the cycle.

Over time you will build enough strength and consistency to maintain your results.

Keep revisiting your "What are you fighting for?" list.

The clearer that purpose becomes, the easier it is to stay on track.

QUANTUM PALEO

"This is my job"

That needs to be your answer to the following questions:

"How did you lose weight?"

"How do you stay in shape?"

"How do you get up and work out before work?"

"How do you do it?"

I want you to start treating health and fitness as if it were your job. It is your job to stay healthy. Isn't that true for you? It has to be. You can't mess around with this. It is a life-or-death situation. You do not need to wait for a heart attack to get inspired.

Your ticket has already been printed with heart disease, Type 2 diabetes, and degenerative illness somewhere in the fine print. The only things you may be able to influence are when and whether. Everyone has the potential to succumb to disease and infirmity. Tear up the ticket. Refuse to give in.

What if you made it your highest priority to live healthy, eat healthy, and exercise consistently with passion? If you choose to make that the priority, you may change the timing and the outcome of your life. Instead of falling apart before your time, choose to live long and age with strength, stamina, and health.

I do not know about you, but when the alarm rings on workdays, I get up immediately. I do not negotiate with myself about whether I am going to work that day.

Why?

Because I have a relationship with my work that is not negotiable. I go to work and do my job. Period. My family needs me. I need food and shelter. It is a matter of survival.

Health has to become the same way.

Raise the stakes. Make it extremely important. That is the trick. That is what you need to know.

With that realization, you take the responsibility of staying well to the highest level.

"I stay healthy because it is my job."

What will it cost you if you gain the weight back?

If you decide this is your job, then it deserves a place in your schedule. A job comes with a schedule. I used to work out only when I had free time. That was planning for failure. As a result, I was overweight, fatigued, depressed, and starting to develop health problems.

Since 2009, I have scheduled workouts into my week. Start doing this. It works.

Monday, Tuesday, Thursday, and Friday I'm at Hell's Kitchen CrossFit from 7:00 to 8:00 a.m. I see my first patients at 9:00 a.m. I get up at 4:45 a.m. to catch a 5:30 a.m. bus into New York City. Door to door it takes me 90 minutes.

I also do three spin classes per week on my lunch break. Then I go to a gym near my house on either Saturday or Sunday with my daughter and do a light workout, stretch, and some cardio. Otherwise, I take long walks with my wife and dogs on the weekends.

This is my job. I schedule it and get it done. I do not consider whether I am in the mood. That is irrelevant. It is not my hobby. It is on my schedule. It needs to get done. It is my job.

As soon as you begin the journey and start chiseling away the debris to reveal the body you want to live in, you must take on this new attitude.

"Of course I exercise."

"Of course I choose healthy foods."

It is simply what I do.

How To Get Off the Roller Coaster

I have done a fair amount of gaining and losing weight throughout my adult life. That is what people call the roller coaster.

You have probably heard that most people lose weight and then gain it back. Sometimes they gain back even more than they lost.

This is going to be a short section.

There are only two solutions.

***Solution #1:** What are you fighting for?*

You need to have your why figured out, written down, and read often. It becomes much more powerful when you see it in writing and return to it regularly. Then, when you share your goals with others, it builds even more momentum.

Tell someone you love that your goal is not just to lose weight, but to keep it off. The why is even more important than the number.

Tell a friend or loved one, *"The reason I am going to keep the weight off is ______."*

"I will keep the weight off because I want to play with my grandkids."

"I will keep the weight off because I want to look amazing in a bathing suit in every decade of my life."

I will keep the weight off because I want a healthy heart."

Solution #2: Exercise

Over the years, whenever I have worked with patients who lose weight without adopting an exercise program, I worry.

I worry because people who do not make exercise part of their lives are far more likely to gain the weight back.

I worry because you are about 75 percent more likely to gain back the weight if you have not made exercise part of your life. Conversely, we can safely say that you are 75 percent more likely to keep it off if you have a vigorous, consistent, and frequent exercise program as part of your weekly routine.

That is it. Do not make it more complicated than it needs to be.

Make it a life-or-death commitment. Because in many ways, it is.

The Acceptable Window

Everyone's weight fluctuates throughout the day. Mine can move three to four pounds in either direction. I might wake up at 187 pounds, for example, and weigh 189 pounds before bed. The next morning I may be 186.8.

That is one type of window. It is the normal daily fluctuation of body weight.

The second window is what I call the Acceptable Window, or the Allowable Window. The Acceptable Window is the weekly range in which your weight is allowed to fluctuate while you are still maintaining your results.

Let's say you started at 176 pounds and after three months on Quantum Paleo you now weigh 150 pounds. My goal for you, and hopefully your goal too, is to maintain those results. No relapse.

To do that, you need to understand your new weekly window.

Let's use a fictional example with someone named Joe Wyndoe.

Let's say we weighed Joe every morning for one week before he started Quantum Paleo.

Every weigh-in is taken first thing in the morning, after using the bathroom, with no clothes on, moments after getting out of bed.

His numbers might look like this:

Monday 175.0 lbs.

Tuesday 176.4 lbs.

Wednesday 174.9 lbs.

Thursday 174.7 lbs.

Friday 174.1 lbs.

Saturday 177.4 lbs.

Sunday 177.9 lbs.

The average would be 175.77 pounds. The average is useful, but the range matters more. Joe's weight fluctuated between 174.1 and 177.9 over the week. That is a swing of 3.8 pounds.

I also like to know body fat percentage at each window. For this example, let's say Joe averages 21.5 percent body fat.

Now let's say three months later Joe loses about 25 pounds on Quantum Paleo. We track him again and find that his weight now moves between 149 and 151.5 pounds in a given week. His body fat percentage is about 15.5 percent. Excellent.

Joe wants to maintain his new body. In the past he always gained the weight back. This time he learns that his new weight naturally fluctuates between 149 and 151.5 pounds. When someone asks what he weighs, he will most likely say, "About 150."

Joe must learn this new window and fight to stay inside it. If he starts drifting up into the 152 to 154 range, that is no longer acceptable. That should trigger immediate action. He needs to analyze his workouts, food choices, bad carbohydrates, fat intake, portion size, sleep, and stress level, and make the necessary corrections.

Fix it. The math is off. Fix the math.

For Joe, the only Acceptable Window is 149 to 151.5 pounds. Period. Know your window. Fight for it.

CrossFit: The Way Our Bodies Were Meant to Train

This past year I changed my training philosophy dramatically. For years I was the typical chest-and-arms guy with a little cardio thrown in. That approach gave me a decent bench press, substantial love handles, a noticeable belly when I was not sucking it in, and mediocre endurance.

I cannot remember whether a patient first recommended CrossFit to me or whether I stumbled across it online. Either way, it became a passion for me.

The following ideas were influenced by Greg Glassman, the founder of CrossFit, who described CrossFit as a core strength and conditioning program designed to develop broad physical competence across many domains of fitness.

CrossFit Journal reference

The basic idea is that true fitness is not about specializing in one narrow skill. It is about becoming capable across multiple physical demands: cardiovascular endurance, stamina, strength, flexibility, power, speed, coordination, agility, balance, and accuracy.

That makes sense to me.

After reading *Starting Strength* by Mark Rippetoe and Lon Kilgore, I also became more convinced than ever that multi-joint exercises and functional movement are the superior way to train the body.

Rippetoe and Kilgore argue that physical strength determines much of the quality and quantity of our time in these bodies. As a health provider, I would add categories like immune function and mental health, but I understand their point.

Take a walk through a hospital or nursing home if you need motivation. Look at the people who have lost their strength. Many can no longer walk, sit up, or feed themselves.

That is one of my biggest fears.

Being trapped in a broken-down body.

Possessing physical strength is foundational to living well in the physical world. The good news is that strength is something we can all work on.

How many hours per day or per week can you commit to your physical health? That is a great question.

Then ask yourself this: what type of exercise is worth that time?

My daughter Lily, for example, has done high school cheerleading. She has had to perform tumbling runs involving back handsprings and flips. At other times she had to lift teammates overhead. Those are all functional movements. They require multiple joints working together under load. They train coordination, balance, strength, speed, and control.

A bicep curl, by contrast, mostly involves one joint.

A big bicep may look impressive, but it does not do much for you in everyday life. My wrestling coach used to tell us that isolated bicep work had very little carryover to sports. He used to say the real engines of performance are the shoulders, back, glutes, trunk, legs, forearms, and grip, along with the posterior chain running along the back of the body.

The part you cannot admire in the mirror.

A squat, which is essentially a deep knee bend with a barbell across your back, involves multiple joints and multiple muscle groups working together. That is how the human body was built to move.

Rippetoe and Kilgore make this point clearly. The body functions as a complete system. It prefers to be trained as a complete system. The pattern of strength acquisition should resemble the pattern in which strength will actually be used.

That makes perfect sense.

If your goal is simply to look good, then single-joint exercises can help. But if your goal is to live long and remain able to run, jump, climb, drag, row, reach, push, pull, twist, and move powerfully through life, then you need functional movement under load.

At this point you may ask, why do I need to do all those things?

Because the inability to do them defines the limitations of your physical life. Imagine not being able to bend down and pick up your grandchild off the floor. All those abilities are either freedoms or limitations. It is your choice which ones you build.

That is one of the reasons I love CrossFit.

The beauty of CrossFit is that it is scalable. The weight, speed, and intensity can all be adjusted to fit the age, sex, size, and ability of the individual. Someone can perform the same movement pattern with a broomstick while another person does it with a loaded barbell.

Different loads. Same movement. Same training principle.

What are you fighting for?

That is the question I ask patients when they are taking on a major health challenge.

What counts as a major challenge?

How about losing the weight you gained over the last decade?

How about balancing your hormones naturally?

How about cutting out grains, sugar, and dairy because you know it is time to get your digestion and inflammation under control?

These goals are difficult because they cannot be achieved overnight.

If I can help people connect with what they are fighting for, that becomes the springboard they need to launch real change. What is the one thing that must change in order for you to reach your goal?

A patient named Deb once came to my office wanting to lose 20 pounds.

Why? I always ask why.

She was getting married in three months. She was 29 years old and had carried extra weight on her hips, abdomen, thighs, and buttocks throughout her adult life. She knew what she was fighting for. Now she needed a how.

The Quantum Paleo program is challenging on its own, but I pushed her harder. I had her do cardio five days per week. She chose three spin classes and two days of walking. She had already been doing one private Pilates session per week, and that was her entire exercise routine.

She liked Pilates, so I encouraged her to continue, but I suggested replacing one expensive private session with more group classes so she could train more often.

By the way, I do not force people to do CrossFit. Everyone gets to choose the training style that fits them best. If I am asked what I recommend, I say CrossFit. In Deb's case, she loved Pilates and spin classes. Fine.

She worked incredibly hard.

She lost 23 pounds. At 5'3", that is a major transformation. Her abdomen flattened, the excess weight on her hips and thighs disappeared, and her face changed dramatically. Her jawline became more defined, her cheekbones became visible, and her overall coloring improved from pale and tired to vibrant.

Three months after her wedding she stabilized her weight and even lost another three pounds. She cut back to three or four days of cardio and two Pilates classes per week. She drinks wine two nights per week. She does not touch bread or pasta during the week. She relaxes a bit one weekend day. Ice cream is for Saturday night only, and she does not keep it in the house.

Her weight fluctuates between 117 and 120 pounds. That is her Acceptable Window. If her weight rises above 120, she immediately gets back on track.

The concept of what are you fighting for is the key to the Quantum Paleo program. You must declare it and make it a priority.

There has to be a conversation going on in your head. You need to recognize the immature voice that does not want to work out, does not want to eat well, and does not want to get off the couch.

That is the four-year-old voice.

Do you really want a four-year-old running your life?

My kids are older now. I was lenient in certain areas as a parent, but when it came to health, education, and safety, I knew how to say no.

The same thing happens in my own mind. I plan to go to the gym. My four-year-old voice says, "Let's skip today."

No. It is not negotiable.

The four-year-old says, "Let's have that cookie now."

No. Eat your protein.

Deb got very good at parenting her own four-year-old voice. She has ice cream, but not every day. She has wine, but not every day. She is the adult. She decides how to live. She made a decision that she will not allow herself to get above 120 pounds. If she does, she responds immediately. She adds cardio. She tightens the diet. It is not negotiable.

I am often asked how I teach people to maintain their desired weight. There are plenty of tips and tricks, but the bottom line is this: know what you are fighting for, and make a pact with yourself that veering too far off course is not negotiable.

Just like Deb.

When you get outside your Acceptable Window, it is hammer time.

Round 9

The Fighters

Meet some fighters

I have been supervising patients through the transition from a grain-heavy diet to a Paleolithic style of eating for 14 years. I have seen approximately 1,800 patients go through this process. While every person's experience is different, I chose a handful of cases that highlight the health potential and possibilities that can exist when switching to a Quantum Paleo lifestyle.

I cannot tell you the patients' real names because there are strict laws protecting personal information. I changed the names and altered identifying details enough to protect their privacy. I did not change the patient history, lab values, or the results.

Hormone Helen

"At 51, I hadn't had my period in 11 months. I was suffering from hot flashes every night. After about two months, it escalated into the daytime too. During the day, I could have six or more hot flashes, and a few of those daytime ones would literally soak through my shirt. I started bringing extra shirts to work. I was embarrassed because I knew people would notice a new shirt in the middle of the day. My diet was off when I met Dr. Willen. I had gained weight over the previous five years and was 17 pounds heavier than I had been at 46 years old. That was the age when everything started slipping.

He put me on his program. We focused on one 21-day round at a time. It took me three rounds of 21 days. Within the first 10 days, my hot flash frequency dropped to nighttime only. Then during my second round of the Quantum Paleo program, I was down to two or three mild hot flashes per week. That's per week, not per day. In my third round of Quantum Paleo, I had one mild hot flash during the entire three weeks.

I have more energy now and my libido returned. I'm sleeping better and getting more total sleep than I have in 10 years. I am making the right choices with my food with very little effort. Dr. Doug told me that exercise would be the stabilizing force, and that is exactly what happened. By making exercise my job, I am not worried about gaining back the weight. One more thing: I used to get a herpes outbreak every few years. Then this past year, it started happening continuously. Dr. Doug said he often sees that kind of thing improve when people shift toward a Paleolithic diet. He was right. That cleared up pretty fast, and I don't feel like it's about to resurface anytime soon. The price of feeling lousy is too high. It is now my highest priority to be healthy. It took me all three rounds, but I finally lost 21 pounds total."

Hearty Arty

"I'm 63 years old and had two stents put in my heart recently. I quit smoking after my heart attack two years ago. I was taking several medications, including prescriptions for cholesterol, blood pressure, and a blood thinner. Although I had already lost 37 pounds, my cardiologist wanted me to lose at least another 30. The problem was that my weight hadn't budged in six months.

I decided to do the Quantum Paleo program. Dr. Doug suggested I join a CrossFit gym near my office, and he put me on Quantum Paleo. I had to stop eating bran muffins, oatmeal, and all the whole grains the hospital dietitian had me eating. That made me nervous. I was also scared about all the fat in the Quantum Paleo program. Dr. Doug told me the blood tests would prove there was no need to worry. He always told me, 'Fat doesn't make you fat,' and 'It's the refined carbohydrate diet that is elevating your blood work, not the avocados, eggs, and olive oil.'

I lost an additional 36 pounds on Quantum Paleo. It took four rounds of 21 days. The most astonishing thing was that my medical doctor was able to take me off my blood pressure medication. My statin is now at the smallest possible dose, reduced by 75 percent. We decided to leave me on Plavix because my cardiologist felt it was too risky to change that one. I have a 32-inch waist now. Same size as in college."

Jay Pouch

"I had my first colon surgery at age 20. After terrible pain, bloating, bloody stools, diarrhea, and recurring bouts of fever for two years, along with numerous hospital visits, my surgeon thought it was time. Over the next 10 years, I needed more surgery. Five more, to be exact. They removed about 95 percent of my large intestine. Eventually they created a J-pouch, which is a pouch typically constructed from the small intestine.

It is also called an ileoanal reservoir procedure. The J-pouch is a storage place for stool that I eventually pass several times per day.

The reason I came to Dr. Willen was that at 31 years old, I was still having problems. Digestion, pain, swelling, gas pockets, adhesions, the list goes on. I was on a long list of medications. Dr. Willen urged me to start the Quantum Paleo diet. First he wanted to confirm his suspicion about gluten and dairy. He ordered a Food Sensitivity (IgG) Test. In the two weeks while we waited for the results, he had me start zero grains, zero dairy, and zero sugar. He said if a patient is in a health crisis, they need to be 100 percent off the three whites, grains, sugar, and dairy. Period. By the time the test came back, I was sleeping through the night. I was reducing my painkillers and anti-inflammatories. I was already feeling better than I had in a long time.

The tests came back with gluten as a major hit. So was dairy and about 10 other foods. All grains lit up positive in the abnormal ranges. It has now been four months, and I really have no symptoms. I was diagnosed with ulcerative colitis, which Dr. Doug said I definitely had. He wanted to know what was causing the ulcerations. He said grains can do that to some people.

My medical team never felt there was a food connection. As far as medicine goes, the cause is unknown and may be related to some foods or a problem with the immune system. The funny thing is that for the last 10 years they wanted me eating a bland diet of pasta, white toast, saltines, noodle soup, and similar foods. I was on a Neolithic agricultural-era diet for the past 10 years. My grain intake was ridiculous. I am so glad I switched from Neo to Paleo."

Goode Knight

"Dr. Doug put me on the Quantum Paleo program about three months ago. At the time I was sleeping about four total hours per night. I seemed to fall asleep pretty well, but I would wake up within one or two hours and then have trouble getting back to sleep. Eventually I would fall asleep again for another two hours, and then after waking up the second time I would not get back to sleep. I always felt this strange buzzing feeling in my body in the middle of the night. It is hard to describe, but the best way I can say it is that it felt like I had a triple shot of espresso at 2 a.m. every night. I was on zero caffeine, by the way.

Dr. Doug explained that all the refined carbohydrates I was addicted to were interfering with my ability to get a good night's sleep. Although he didn't promise anything, he was grinning when he said, 'Let's wait and see.'

Meanwhile, I needed to lose some weight anyway, and I had a few other things I was dealing with, including chronic aches and pains. After about 15 days, I was sleeping through the night. Only about 6.5 hours at first, but then eventually 7.5 to 8 hours. Dr. Doug suggested that I black out my room, move all electrical devices out of the room, and start going to sleep an hour earlier.

I think a big part of it was getting my health and diet corrected. My aches and pains have reduced by 85 percent. I also lost eight pounds in the first three weeks and a total of 22 pounds, and I'm maintaining."

Mike Bladher

"I had been a college basketball player and continued to play in competitive men's leagues throughout my adult life. I ate well, lifted weights, and played basketball several times per week. My waist was still 34 inches.

Then at 49, I was urinating after watching a movie with my wife and kids when dark blood came out with my urine. I was terrified. To make a long story shorter, a week later I was diagnosed with bladder cancer.

Surgery was scheduled within a few weeks. It was a major procedure. They were afraid the cancer was aggressive and may have already spread. My prognosis was not good. I went to Dr. Doug to have him look at my diet.

He told me that if he were in my shoes, he would get his diet as clean as possible before surgery. He said, 'We need to get you in fighting shape.' That way you become the best possible candidate to create a miracle. He wanted me to eliminate the three whites: grains, dairy, and sugar. I thought my diet was already pretty good. He wanted me to go off all flour and grains, and also totally stop dairy and sugar. I had never done this before because I always thought athletes needed plenty of healthy grains and several glasses of milk every day. I tried to negotiate with him. I wanted him to allow a little whole grain and at least one glass of milk per day. He said, '100 percent compliance or don't bother starting.' I decided to follow the rules. I did the diet perfectly. I approached it like a fight for my life.

(Note: This story was from 2002. I didn't have the word Paleo in my vocabulary back then. I called it getting off the three whites.)

The surgery went well. My medical team bragged about how fast I recovered. It has now been two years. Cancer free. I still eat this way. I now have a 32-

inch waist, play basketball several times per week, and my immune system feels very strong. I never get sick anymore. I sleep like a baby. My allergies have disappeared. I could go on, but I think you get the idea."

(Note: Mike is still very healthy, cancer free, and eating a Paleo diet.)

Al Kohol

"I was abusing alcohol through most of my 20s, and by 35 it was getting worse. My career and marriage went down the drain. I was 50 pounds overweight and looked like I was in my late 40s. Alcohol really destroys the skin and ages you rapidly.

I met Dr. Doug after being sober for four weeks. My sponsor in AA was a patient of his and told me to get checked.

Dr. Doug offers all of his patients an opportunity to get on program. That means he gets your diet cleaned up and gives you a routine of daily supplements to address deficiencies and help build health naturally. I thought I might benefit from getting on a health-building program to offset the destroy-my-body program I had been on for years.

I was thinking about drinking every day. All day long, actually. I felt like I might slip. I was even dreaming most nights that I had relapsed and gone on a binge, only to wake up and realize it was just a vivid dream. I was scared. On top of that, I gained another 15 pounds in those first four weeks off alcohol. I was eating bread, sugar, sweets, desserts, potato chips, pretzels, and especially bagels. Bagels for breakfast. Tuna on a bagel at lunch. I was craving bread like an addict.

Dr. Doug put me on the Quantum Paleo program. In addition, he did his weird-arm testing, what he calls nutritional kinesiology. That is where he figures out what nutrients and supplements a person needs to reclaim their health. I call it weird-arm testing, but I have to admit it really works.

Within three days, my sugar cravings were gone. I was off bread. My bloated face and belly started to reduce. Dr. Doug wanted me to do cardio six days per week and weights three times per week. I lost 22 pounds the first month. After three months, I was down 42 pounds. After six months, I had lost a total of 72 pounds. I was stable in my sobriety. I no longer felt vulnerable to relapse. I was in a new relationship. I started a new career in a whole new direction. Actually, it was the work I had always wanted to do, but never felt confident enough to pursue.

Dr. Doug explained to me that getting off grains and sugar, in my case, would help tremendously with my addiction. Not only was I addicted to alcohol, but he said my carbohydrate addiction was adding gasoline to the fire."

ROUND 10

WRAP UP

Resources

The following resources may help you continue learning about nutrition, health, and lifestyle after finishing this book.

Websites and Educational Resources

RobbWolf.com

Robb Wolf's work on Paleo nutrition and lifestyle.

MarksDailyApple.com

Mark Sisson's widely read website on ancestral health and the Primal lifestyle.

ThePaleoDiet.com

Dr. Loren Cordain's website and research on Paleolithic nutrition.

Whole9Life.com

A resource focused on whole foods nutrition and lifestyle habits.

EatWild.com

Information about sourcing grass fed and naturally raised animal foods.

SeafoodWatch.org

The Monterey Bay Aquarium's guide to sustainable seafood choices.

DrCate.com

Dr. Cate Shanahan's writing on nutrition, metabolism, and traditional foods.

Cookbooks

The Primal Blueprint Cookbook by Mark Sisson

Everyday Paleo by Sarah Fragoso

The Paleo Diet Cookbook by Loren Cordain

Recommended Reading

The Paleo Diet by Loren Cordain

The Paleo Solution by Robb Wolf

Wheat Belly by William Davis

Why We Get Fat by Gary Taubes

Dangerous Grains by James Braly and Ron Hoggan

The Primal Blueprint by Mark Sisson

Primal Body, Primal Mind by Nora Gedgaudas

Pandora's Seed by Spencer Wells

Round 11

Still Fighting

When I first wrote Quantum Paleo, I was in the middle of a personal fight.

A fight to reclaim my health, my energy, and my body.

The ideas in this book came from years of working with patients and experimenting on myself. Real food. Hard training. Discipline. Getting back to the basics that the human body was designed for.

At the time, the idea of removing grains, sugar, and processed foods felt radical to many people. Today it has become far more common. What was once considered extreme is now widely discussed in mainstream health circles.

Fifteen years later, the core principles of this book still hold true.

Real food matters.

Strength and movement matter.

Consistency matters.

The modern world has not made these things easier. If anything, the environment around us has become even more challenging. Processed food is everywhere. Many people sleep poorly, sit too much, and live under constant stress.

The fight for health is still very real.

Over the years I have had the opportunity to watch thousands of people transform their health through simple changes in diet, exercise, and lifestyle. I have also learned something important since writing the original version of this book.

Food and exercise are powerful tools.

But they are not the entire picture.

There is another system in the body that quietly influences almost every aspect of health. It affects sleep, metabolism, stress levels, hormone balance, recovery, and even body weight.

Breathing.

When we breathe well, the body functions more efficiently. When breathing is dysfunctional, the entire system begins to struggle.

This realization opened a new chapter in my work and research. I began studying breathing patterns, sleep, airway health, and the connection between breathing and overall wellness.

What I discovered reinforced something I already believed.

The human body responds powerfully when we return to simple fundamentals.

Eat real food.

Move your body.

Sleep deeply.

Breathe properly.

Reduce unnecessary stress.

Spend time outdoors.

Build strength.

Connect with people.

These principles may sound simple, but simple does not mean easy. The world we live in constantly pulls us away from these foundations.

That is why the metaphor of fighting is still appropriate.

Health is not something you fix once and then forget about.

It is something you defend.

Round after round.

Some rounds are easy. You are motivated, focused, and disciplined.

Other rounds are harder. Life becomes busy. Stress creeps in. Old habits try to return.

The key is not perfection.

The key is staying in the fight.

Every meal is a small decision.

Every workout is a small decision.

Every night of good sleep is a small victory.

Those decisions accumulate over time and shape the direction of your life.

You may not be able to control every health challenge that appears in your life. But you can control how you respond to them.

You can decide what you are fighting for.

You can decide how you train, how you eat, how you move, and how you care for your body.

You can decide that your health is worth protecting.

That is the spirit behind Quantum Paleo.

It was never meant to be a short term diet or a temporary program. It was meant to be a reset. A way of returning to the fundamentals that help human beings thrive.

If this book helped you start that process, then it has done its job.

The rest of the journey belongs to you.

Keep learning.

Keep training.

Keep questioning what the modern world tells you about health.

And most importantly, keep fighting.

Because your future health will not be decided in a single moment.

It will be decided round by round, choice by choice, day by day.

Stay in the fight.

FINAL THOUGHTS

"Let others lead small lives, but not you. Let others argue over small things, but not you. Let others cry over small hurts, but not you. Let others leave their future in someone else's hands, but not you."

Jim Rohn

The late Jim Rohn was one of my mentors. I never met him, but I listened to his tapes and read his books over and over again. My final thoughts are woven around two of my favorite Jim Rohn quotes as a way to pay homage to this great inspirational teacher.

Losing weight and improving your health can become a catalyst for change in every area of your life. Sometimes we all feel as if our circumstances are so overwhelming that we do not know where to start. All change starts at the core. Change the way you eat. Change the way you exercise, and your world will change.

Decide what is worth fighting for, and go change your world.

"You cannot change your destination overnight, but you can change your direction overnight."

Jim Rohn

About Dr. Doug

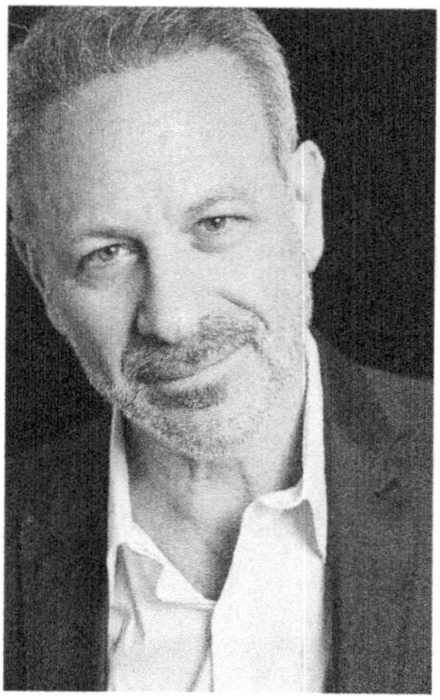

A chiropractor saved me from being benched from sports in high school by taking what seemed like a hopeless injury and turning it around. That was my first exposure to the power of natural solutions for health. While my family medical doctor could only offer pain medication and restrictions, the chiropractor offered a path to recovery. That experience left a lasting impression and ultimately shaped my career.

At the time I was a pre-med student at Cornell University. My experiences with natural health care and my own struggles with allergies led me to question the heavy pharmaceutical focus of conventional medicine. I began working with alternative practitioners who were interested in understanding the root causes of health problems rather than simply suppressing symptoms. For the first time I experienced meaningful improvement.

After graduating from Cornell, I spent nearly two years traveling throughout India, Asia, and Central America. Living among local communities and observing different cultural approaches to health, food, and spirituality had a profound influence on me. That time shaped my understanding of how lifestyle, diet, and mindset affect long term health.

When I returned to the United States, I pursued my goal of becoming a natural health practitioner and attended Life University in Atlanta, where I earned my Doctorate in Chiropractic.

I eventually returned to New York and opened a chiropractic and nutrition practice in New York City. During this period I studied nutritional kinesiology with one of the pioneers in the field, Fred Ulan. Dr. Ulan later entrusted me with the care of his long standing New York City patients. It was an honor to be his protégé and to continue helping the people he had served for many years.

My practice focused on helping people rebuild their health through natural strategies including nutrition, lifestyle changes, targeted supplementation, and expert chiropractic care. Much of the practice grew through word of mouth referrals. When people improved their health they often sent their friends and family members to my office.

Over the years I worked with a diverse range of people including performers from the Broadway community, dancers, actors, musicians, athletes, and professionals from many industries. Helping people rebuild their health from the inside out became the foundation of my approach.

The Quantum Paleo program grew directly out of that work. Over many years of clinical practice I observed how powerful dietary changes could be when people removed processed foods and refined carbohydrates and focused on real, whole foods combined with consistent exercise and lifestyle improvements.

Quantum Paleo is the result of those years of experience helping patients transform their health and their bodies.

The Journey Continues

If this book sparked something in you, the journey does not end here.

Over the years my work has continued to evolve. What began with nutrition and lifestyle eventually expanded into breathing, sleep, and airway health. These areas play a powerful role in energy, metabolism, recovery, and long term health.

If you would like to continue learning, I invite you to visit:

ExhaleMethod.com

There you will find additional resources, training programs, and educational material designed to help you improve your breathing, sleep, and overall health.

Scan the QR code below to continue the journey.

www.exhalemethod.com

Inside you will find:

The Exhale Method Masterclass

The Breathing Gym

Apnea Unmasked

Additional resources for improving breathing, sleep, and metabolic health.

Keep fighting for your health.

Dr. Doug

Selected References

- Andersen, H. C., Edgar Lucas, H. B. Paull, and Arthur Szyk. *Andersen's Fairy Tales.* New York: Grosset & Dunlap, 1945. Print.
- Appleton, Nancy. *Lick the Sugar Habit.* Garden City Park, NY: Avery Pub. Group, 1996. Print.
- Astrup, A., and J. Dyerberg. "The Role of Reducing Intakes of Saturated Fat in the Prevention of Cardiovascular Disease: Where Does the Evidence Stand in 2010." *Am Journal of Clinical Nutrition.* 4th ser. 93. April (2011): 684-8. Print.
- Balch, Phyllis A., and James F. Balch. *Prescription for Nutritional Healing.* New York: Avery, 2000. Print.
- Ballentine, Rudolph. *Diet and Nutrition a Holistic Approach.* Honesdale, Pa: Himalayan International Institute, 1979. Print.
- Batmanghelidj, F. *Your Body's Many Cries for Water.* [S.l.]: Tagman, 2004. Print.
- Borhanihaghighi, A., N. Ansari, M. Mokhtari, B. Geramizadeh, and K. Lankarani. "Multiple Sclerosis and Gluten Sensitivity☆." *Clinical Neurology and Neurosurgery.* 109.8 (2007): 651-53. Print.
- Braly, James, and Ron Hoggan. *Dangerous Grains: Why Gluten Cereal Grains May Be Hazardous to Your Health.* New York: Avery, 2002. Print.
- Briani, C., D. Samaroo, and A. Alaedini. "Celiac Disease: From Gluten to Autoimmunity." *Autoimmunity Reviews.* 7.8 (2008): 644-50. Print.

- Brody, Julia Green, Ruthann A. Rudel, Karin B. Michels, and Kirsten B. Moysich. "Environmental Pollutants, Diet, Physical Activity, Body Size, and Breast Cancer." *Cancer.* 109.S12 (2007): 2627-634. Print.
- Case, Shelley. *Gluten-free Diet: A Comprehensive Resource Guide.* Regina: Case Nutrition Consulting, 2002. Print.
- Challem, Jack, Burt Berkson, and Melissa Diane Smith. *Syndrome X: The Complete Nutritional Program to Prevent and Reverse Insulin Resistance.* New York: Wiley, 2000. Print.
- Chevat, Richie, and Michael Pollan. *The Omnivore's Dilemma: The Secrets behind What You Eat.* New York: Dial, 2009. Print.
- Cohen, Mark Nathan. *Health and the Rise of Civilization.* New Haven: Yale UP, 1989. Print.
- Collin, Pekka, and Timo Reunala. "Recognition and Management of the Cutaneous Manifestations of Celiac Disease." *American Journal of Clinical Dermatology.* 4.1 (2003): 13-20. Print.
- Cordain, Loren. "Introduction." *The Paleo Diet: Lose Weight and Get Healthy by Eating the Food You Were Designed to Eat.* New York: Wiley, 2003. 3-7. Print.
- Crawford, Michael A., Richard P. Bazinet, and Andrew J. Sinclair. "Fat Intake and CNS Functioning: Ageing and Disease." *Annals of Nutrition and Metabolism.* 55.1-3 (2009): 202-28. Print.
- Crawford, Michael, and David Marsh. *The Nutrition and Evolution.* New Canaan, CT: Keats Publ., 1995. Print.
- Croft, N. "IgG Food Antibodies and Irritating the Bowel." *Gastroenterology.* 128.4 (2005): 1135-136. Print.

- Davis, William, and John A. Rumberger. *Track Your Plaque: The Only Heart Disease Prevention Program That Shows You How to Use the New Heart Scans to Detect, Track, and Control Coronary Plaque.* New York: iUniverse, 2004. Print.
- De Lorgeril, Michel, Patricia Salen, Jean-Louis Martin, François Boucher, and Joël De Leiris. "Interactions of Wine Drinking with Omega-3 Fatty Acids in Patients with Coronary Heart Disease: A Fish-like Effect of Moderate Wine Drinking." *American Heart Journal.* 155.1 (2008): 175-81. Print.
- Della Valle, N., S. Prencipe, and V. De Francesco. "P.208 Body Composition And Dietary Intakes In Adult Coeliac Disease Patients From Southern Italy Consuming A Strict Gluten-Free Diet." *Digestive and Liver Disease.* 42 (2010): S175. Print.
- Diamond, Jared M. *The Third Chimpanzee: The Evolution and Future of the Human Animal.* New York: HarperPerennial, 2006. Print.
- Dickey, William, and Natalie Kearney. "Overweight in Celiac Disease: Prevalence, Clinical Characteristics, and Effect of a Gluten-Free Diet." *The American Journal of Gastroenterology.* 101.10 (2006): 2356-359. Print.
- Docena, G. H., R. Fernandez, F. G. Chirdo, and C. A. Fossati. "Identification of Casein as the Major Allergenic and Antigenic Protein of Cow's Milk." *Allergy.* 51.6 (1996): 412-16. Print.
- Donnelly, Joseph E., Bryan Smith, Dennis J. Jacobsen, Erik Kirk, Katrina DuBose, Melissa Hyder, Bruce Bailey, and Richard Washburn. "The Role of Exercise for Weight Loss and Maintenance." *Best Practice & Research Clinical Gastroenterology.* 18.6 (2004): 1009-029. Print.
- Dorland, W. A. Newman. *Dorland's Medical Dictionary.* Philadelphia, PA: Saunders, 1980. Print.

- Eades, Michael R., and Mary Dan. Eades. *Protein Power: The High Protein, Low Carbohydrate Way to Lose Weight, Feel Fit, and Boost Your Health.* London: Thorsons, 2000. Print.
- Eades, Michael R., and Mary Dan. Eades. *Protein Power: The Metabolic Breakthrough.* New York: Bantam, 1996. Print.
- Eaton, S. Boyd, and Melvin Konner. "Paleolithic Nutrition." *The New England Journal of Medicine.* 312.5 (1985): 283-89. Print.
- Elder, Jennifer Harrison, Meena Shankar, and Jonathan Shuster. "The Gluten-Free, Casein-Free Diet In Autism: Results of A Preliminary Double Blind Clinical Trial." *Journal of Autism and Developmental Disorders.* Print. Disorders. 36.3 (2006): 413-20. Print.
- "The Emperor's New Clothes." *Wikipedia.* Accessed December 30, 2011. http://en.wikipedia.org/wiki/The_Emperor's_New_Clothes.
- Enig, Mary G. *Know Your Fats: The Complete Primer for Understanding the Nutrition of Fats, Oils and Cholesterol.* Silver Spring, MD: Bethesda, 2000. Print.
- Erasmus, Udo. *Fats That Heal, Fats That Kill: The Complete Guide to Fats, Oils, Cholesterol, and Human Health.* Burnaby, BC, Canada: Alive, 1993. Print.
- Frost, Robert. *Mountain Interval.* New York: H. Holt and, 1921. Print.
- Fuehrlein, B. S. "Differential Metabolic Effects of Saturated Versus Polyunsaturated Fats in Ketogenic Diets." *Journal of Clinical Endocrinology & Metabolism.* 89.4 (2004): 1641-645. Print.

- Gannon, M. C., and F. Q. Nuttall. "Effect of a High-Protein, Low-Carbohydrate Diet on Blood Glucose Control in People With Type 2 Diabetes." *Diabetes.* 53.9 (2004): 2375-382. Print.
- Gittleman, Ann Louise. *The Fat Flush Plan.* New York: McGraw-Hill, 2002. Print.
- Glassman, Greg. "Nutrition: An Interview With Fast Company Magazine." *CrossFit Journal.* Fast Track Magazine Exclusive Interview, 11 Oct. 2011. Web. http://journal.crossfit.com/2011/10/greggasmnutrition.tpl.
- Goldfinger, T. "Beyond the French Paradox: The Impact of Moderate Beverage Alcohol and Wine Consumption in the Prevention of Cardiovascular Disease." *Cardiology Clinics.* 21.3 (2003): 449-57. Print.
- Guyton, Arthur C., and John E. Hall. *Textbook of Medical Physiology.* Philadelphia: Saunders, 2000. Print.
- Hadjivassiliou, Marios, David S. Sanders, Richard A. Grünewald, Nicola Woodroofe, Sabrina Boscolo, and Daniel Aeschlimann. "Gluten Sensitivity: From Gut to Brain." *The Lancet Neurology.* 9.3 (2010): 318-30. Print.
- Hays, J. H. "The Hunter-Gatherer Diet." *Mayo Clinic Proceedings.* 79 (5) May (2004): 703-04. Print.
- Heaton, K. "Sugar Consumption And Myocardial Infarction." *The Lancet.* 297.7691 (1971): 185-86. Print.
- Horne, J. "Obesity and Short Sleep: Unlikely Bedfellows?" *Obesity Reviews.* (2011): No. Print.
- Hunt, Charles. *Charles Hunt's Diet Evolution: Eat Fat and Get Fit!* Beverly Hills, CA: Maximum Human Potential Productions, 1999. Print.

- Hutchinson, Ezzie. "Celiac Disease: Increased Celiac Disease in IBS." *Nature Reviews Gastroenterology & Hepatology.* 6.7 (2009): 381. Print.
- Ivy, John L. "Role of Exercise Training in the Prevention and Treatment of Insulin Resistance and Non-Insulin-Dependent Diabetes Mellitus." *Sports Medicine.* 24.5 (1997): 321-36. Print.
- Kalaydjian, A. E., W. Eaton, N. Cascella, and A. Fasano. "The Gluten Connection: The Association between Schizophrenia and Celiac Disease." *Acta Psychiatrica Scandinavica.* 113.2 (2006): 82-90. Print.
- Kaufmann, Doug A., and Beverly Thornhill. Hunt. *The Fungus Link: An Introduction to Fungal Disease including the Initial Phase Diet.* Rockwall, TX: MediaTrition, 2000. Print.
- Kaufmann, Doug A., and Beverly Thornhill. Hunt. *The Germ That Causes Cancer: With the Initial Phase Diet, Cancer Edition.* Rockwall, TX: MediaTrition, 2002. Print.
- Kaufmann, Doug A., and David Holland. *What Makes Bread Rise?: A Science-based Weight Loss Program for America's Families.* Rockwall, TX: MediaTrition, 2004. Print.
- Lee, Richard B., and Richard Heywood Daly. *The Cambridge Encyclopedia of Hunters and Gatherers.* Cambridge, U.K.: Cambridge UP, 1999. Print.
- Lefebvre, and Scheen. "Glucose Metabolism and the Postprandial State." *European Journal of Clinical Investigation.* 29.S2. (1999): 1-6. Print.
- Lieberman, Shari, and Linda Segall. *The Gluten Connection: How Gluten Sensitivity May Be Sabotaging Your Health—and What You Can Do to Take Control Now.* [Emmaus, Penn.]: Rodale, 2007. Print.

- Lipski, Elizabeth. *Digestive Wellness: Strengthen the Immune System and Prevent Disease through Healthy Digestion.* New York, NY: McGraw-Hill, 2012. Print.
- Liska, DeAnn, and Jeffrey Bland. *Clinical Nutrition: A Functional Approach.* Gig Harbor, WA: Institute for Functional Medicine, 2004. Print.
- Lorenzen, J. "Gluten-Sensitive Enteropathy And Eczema." *The Lancet.* 285.7388 (1965): 766. Print.
- Ludwig, D., K. Peterson, and S. Gortmaker. "Relation between Consumption of Sugar-sweetened Drinks and Childhood Obesity: A Prospective, Observational Analysis." *The Lancet.* 357.9255 (2001): 505-08. Print.
- Marshall, N., N. Glozier, and R. Grunstein. "Is Sleep Duration Related to Obesity? A Critical Review of the Epidemiological Evidence." *Sleep Medicine Reviews.* 12.4 (2008): 289-98. Print.
- McClenaghan, Neville H. "Determining the Relationship between Dietary Carbohydrate Intake and Insulin Resistance." *Nutrition Research Reviews.* 18.02 (2005): 222. Print.
- Melanson, Edward L., Arne Astrup, and William T. Donahoo. "The Relationship between Dietary Fat and Fatty Acid Intake and Body Weight, Diabetes, and the Metabolic Syndrome." *Annals of Nutrition and Metabolism.* 55.1-3 (2009): 229-43. Print.
- Melnik, Bodo C. "Milk – The Promoter of Chronic Western Diseases." *Medical Hypotheses.* 72.6 (2009): 631-39. Print.
- Moneret Vautrin, D. A., J. Sainte-Laudy, and G. Kanny. "Ulcerative Colitis Possibly Due to Hypersensitivity to Wheat and Egg." *Allergy.* 56.5 (2001): 458-59. Print.

- Niewinski, M. "Advances in Celiac Disease and Gluten-Free Diet." *Journal of the American Dietetic Association.* 108.4 (2008): 661-72. Print.
- Null, Gary. *Nutrition and the Mind.* New York: Four Walls Eight Windows, 1995. Print.
- "Nutrition, Insulin, Insulin-like Growth Factors and Cancer." *Hormone and Metabolic Research.* 35.11/12 (2003): 694-704. Print.
- Parker, G., N. A. Gibson, H. Brotchie, G. Heruc, A.-M. Rees, and D. Hadzi-Pavlovic. "Omega-3 Fatty Acids and Mood Disorders." *American Journal of Psychiatry.* 163.6 (2006): 969-78. Print.
- Patel, Sanjay R., and Frank B. Hu. "Short Sleep Duration and Weight Gain: A Systematic Review." *Obesity.* 16.3 (2008): 643-53. Print.
- Percheron, C. "Metabolic Responses to High Carbohydrate Breakfasts in Obese Patients with Impaired Glucose Tolerance. Comparison of Meals Containing Dairy Products and Fruits versus Bread." *Nutrition Research.* 17.5 (1997): 797-806. Print.
- Pert, Candace B. *Molecules of Emotion.* New York: Scribner, 2003. Pesk in, Brian, and Marcus Conyers. *Beyond the Zone.* Houston, TX: Noble Pub., 2000. Print.
- "Phytate And Rickets." *Nutrition Reviews.* 31.8 (1973): 238-39. Print.
- Pottenger, Francis M., Elaine Pottenger, and Robert T. Pottenger. *Pottenger's Cats: A Study in Nutrition.* La Mesa, CA (P.O. Box 2614, La Mesa 92041): Price-Pottenger Nutrition Foundation, 2009. Print.

- Price, Weston. *Nutrition and Physical Degeneration: A Comparison of Primitive and Modern Diets and Their Effects.* (Hardback). Garsington: Benediction Classics, 2010. Print.
- Ray, Sondra. *The Only Diet There Is.* Berkeley, CA: Celestial Arts, 1981. Print.
- Rippetoe, Mark, and Lon Kilgore. *Starting Strength: Basic Barbell Training.* Wichita Falls, TX: Aasgaard, 2007. Print.
- Robinson, Jo. *Pasture Perfect: The Far-reaching Benefits of Choosing Meat, Eggs, and Dairy Products from Grass-fed Animals.* Vashon, WA: Vashon Island, 2004. Print.
- Ross, Julia. *The Mood Cure: The 4-step Program to Rebalance Your Emotional Chemistry and Rediscover Your Natural Sense of Well-being.* New York: Viking, 2002. Print.
- Roznyek, P., and I. Sander. "TPIS - an IgE-binding Wheat Protein." *Allergy.* 57.5 (2002): 463. Print.
- Ryan, Alice S. "Exercise in Aging: Its Important Role in Mortality, Obesity and Insulin Resistance." *Aging Health.* 6.5 (2010): 551-63. Print.
- Ryan, Frank. *The Eskimo Diet: How to Avoid a Heart Attack.* Ebury Press, 1990. Print.
- Schmid, Ronald F. *The Untold Story of Milk: The History, Politics and Science of Nature's Perfect Food: Raw Milk from Pasture-fed Cows.* Washington, DC: NewTrends Pub., 2009. Print.
- Sears, Barry. *The Zone.* New York: HarperCollins, 1995. Print.
- Shakespeare, William. *Romeo and Juliet.* Act II., Sc. II ed. Oxford, Eng.: Oxford UP., 2002. Print.
- Simopoulos, A. P. "Omega 3 Fatty Acids in the Prevention-management of Cardiovascular Disease." *Can J Physiol Pharmacol.* 1997.75 (1997): 234-9. Print.

- Sinatra, Stephen T., James Roberts, and Martin Zucker. *Reverse Heart Disease Now: Stop Deadly Cardiovascular Plaque before It's Too Late.* Hoboken, NJ: John Wiley & Sons, 2007. Print.
- Sivak, M. "Sleeping More as a Way to Lose Weight." *Obesity Reviews.* 7.3 (2006): 295-96. Print.
- Soleas, George J., Eleftherios P. Diamandis, and David M. Goldberg. "Wine as a Biological Fluid: History, Production, and Role in Disease Prevention." *Journal of Clinical Laboratory Analysis.* 11.5 (1997): 287-313. Print.
- Speth, John D. "Early Hominid Hunting and Scavenging: The Role of Meat as an Energy Source." *Journal of Human Evolution.* 18.4 (1989): 329-43. Print.
- Spiegel, K. "Sleep Loss: A Novel Risk Factor for Insulin Resistance and Type 2 Diabetes." *Journal of Applied Physiology.* 99.5 (2005): 2008-019. Print.
- Stanford, Craig B. *The Hunting Apes: Meat Eating and the Origins of Human Behavior.* Princeton, NJ: Princeton UP, 1999. Print.
- Stockman, J.a. "The Effects of Low-Carbohydrate Versus Conventional Weight Loss Diets in Severely Obese Adults: One-Year Follow-up of a Randomized Trial." *Yearbook of Pediatrics.* 2006 (2006): 428-31. Print.
- Tatham, A. S., and P. R. Shewry. "Allergy to Wheat and Related Cereals." *Clinical & Experimental Allergy.* (2008). Print.
- Tau, C., C. Mautalen, and S. De Rosa. "Bone Mineral Density in Children with Celiac Disease. Effect of a Gluten-free Diet." *European Journal of Clinical Nutrition.* 60.3 (2005): 358-63. Print.

- Tsatsouline, Pavel. *The Naked Warrior: Master the Secrets of the Super-strong, Using Bodyweight Exercises Only.* St. Paul, MN: Dragon Door, 2004. Print.
- Van Cauter, E., and K. L. Knutson. "Sleep and the Epidemic of Obesity in Children and Adults." *European Journal of Endocrinology.* 159.Suppl_1 (2008): S59-66. Print.
- Walford, Roy L. *The 120-year Diet: How to Double Your Vital Years.* New York: Simon and Schuster, 1986. Print.
- Werlinger, Kelly, Teresa K. King, Matthew M. Clark, Vincent Pera, and John P. Wincze. "Perceived Changes in Sexual Functioning and Body Image following Weight Loss in an Obese Female Population: A Pilot Study." *Journal of Sex & Marital Therapy.* 23.1 (1997): 74-78. Print.
- Wilson, James L. *Adrenal Fatigue: The 21st Century Stress Syndrome.* Petaluma, CA: Smart Publications, 2001. Print.
- Wolf, Robb. *The Paleo Solution: The Original Human Diet.* Las Vegas: Victory Belt, 2010. Print.
- Zimmet, P., and C. R. Thomas. "Genotype, Obesity, and Cardiovascular Disease: Has Technical and Social Advancement Outstripped Evolution?" *Journal of Internal Medicine.* 2nd ser. Aug.254 (2003): 114-25. Print.
- Zipes, Jack. *Hans Christian Andersen: The Misunderstood Storyteller.* New York: Routledge, 2005. Print.

Made in the USA
Monee, IL
04 November 2026

67378310R10098